THE CLINICAL EXPERIENCE

The Clinical Experience

The construction and reconstruction of medical reality

PAUL ATKINSON
University College, Cardiff

Gower

Published by
Gower Publishing Co. Ltd.
Westmead, Farnborough, Hampshire, England

British Library Cataloguing in Publication Data

Atkinson, Paul
  The clinical experience.
  1. Social medicine
  2. Diagnosis
  I. Title
  301.5'5   RA418

ISBN 0 566 00413 5

Printed in Great Britain by
Biddles Ltd, Guildford, Surrey

Contents

Acknowledgements

This short monograph is based on part of my Ph D thesis. The original
thesis took several years to complete, and for various reasons, this
book has had to wait several more years to see the light of day. Over
the years a great many people have contributed their help, advice and
encouragement. Among them are Professor Liam Hudson and Peter
Sheldrake, who supervised the original postgraduate work; Professors
A. S. Duncan and H. J. Walton, who eased my passage into the medical
school; Margaret Reid, who shared the experience of research on
medical education; my fellow students and colleagues at Edinburgh,
Stirling and Cardiff. The greatest debt, for colleagueship and
companionship, I owe to Sara Delamont. I have not always taken her
advice, but I almost invariably wish I had.

My research on medical education was originally supported by a
postgraduate studentship from the Social Science Research Council,
and subsequently by a grant from the Nuffield Foundation.

Finally I should like to thank Val Dobie, who has had the unenviable
task of preparing the typescript for this book.

1 The Clinical Tradition

INTRODUCTION

The setting is a hospital ward of unmistakably nineteenth century
origins. In a large open ward a number of patients are sitting up in
bed, more or less comfortable. A number of nurses are bustling about,
dressed in a bewildering variety of colours and styles of uniforms.
There are a few ancillary workers coming in and out of the wards; a
portable X-ray machine is wheeled in, and a patient is wheeled out.
A physiotherapist is looking for her patient, but she has apparently
disappeared, and the therapist acknowledges defeat and leaves. The
furniture and equipment on the ward is modern, but shabby and looks
uncared for. The paintwork manages to be simultaneously fresh and drab.
There is little here to invoke the wonders of modern high technology
medicine, nor yet to provoke anxiety. There is certainly no drama, no
heroics. The patients appear listless, preoccupied with their own
solitude rather than suffering.

Into this ward comes a small group of men and women, all wearing white
coats. Most of them are in their early twenties: an older man is
clearly in charge. Whereas the youngsters seem unsure of themselves, he
enters the ward with an easy air of self assurance. He radiates
authority. They group together at the door and mutter together
conspiratorially, occasionally throwing glances at the occupant of a
bed. The patients and the staff take little notice of the intrusion, it
seems. Most of them are well used to these incursions. We are in a
teaching hospital, and a teaching 'round' is in progress. A consultant
physician is taking a small group of medical students to talk to and
examine one or more of his patients in the ward.

The huddle breaks up, the physician and his students make their way
towards one particular bed. They form themselves into a new group
round the patient; the consultant stands at the head of the bed, to
the patient's right and the students range below him on both sides of
the bed. The screens are pulled round the huddle, and the patient is
entirely hidden behind curtains and bodies.

The patient herself is a skinny woman, with coarse, iron grey hair and
a sallow complexion. The consultant introduces her to the students.
She is sixty two years old, and has been complaining of breathlessness,
but presents no other complaints. She appears not to be in any
distress, nor to be in any way discomfited by the appearance of the
doctor and students.

The consultant turns to one of the students and asks him to start
examining the patient. 'What systems would you want to examine in
relation to Mrs. Baxter's breathlessness?' 'The cardiovascular system
...and the respiratory', the student replies.

'What about anaemia?'

'I was including that in the cardiovascular, 'cos blood goes through that....'

The other students and the doctor chuckle at this apparent gaffe, while its perpetrator looks ashamed and embarrassed. He then begins to examine the patient. Meanwhile a couple of the other students have picked up the patient's chart which was hanging at the foot of the bed. The consultant spots them and they are scolded, 'You'll be able to tell what's wrong with her just by looking at the treatment she's getting'. And so the teaching continues. The students take turns at examining the patient, questioning her and responding to questions from the doctor. The patient replies when she is spoken to, but otherwise takes no active part in the proceedings. She is a compliant 'lay figure'.

That brief description of a round in an Edinburgh teaching hospital would, I assume, come as no surprise to anyone. Even if it is not something one had experienced, from one or other side of the bedclothes, it is part and parcel of our stock of knowledge of how doctors are trained. It is an archetype, just like the 'family doctor' taking a pulse, or the school teacher lecturing in front of a blackboard.

It is this archetype which forms the theme of this monograph, which is addressed to the 'clinical' in undergraduate medical education. It is based on a two year period of participant observation in the Edinburgh medical school, during which I observed 'bedside teaching' in medicine and surgery during the students' first year of clinical studies. The setting and conduct of that research is reported in detail elsewhere (Atkinson, 1976) and space precludes a full account of it here. What is presented in this book is a highly selective account of just one aspect of that ethnographic study: the social construction and reconstruction of medical reality (cf. Berger and Luckmann, 1967; Atkinson, 1977).

I have no intention of attempting to produce a comprehensive account of the socialisation process, of how medical students 'become' doctors. My research was not a longitudinal study of cohorts of students, and in any event the notion of 'socialisation' is highly problematic in this context (Olesen and Whittaker, 1970; Dingwall, 1977). Rather, I concentrate on one particular, crucial phase within the undergraduate course at one medical school. That is, the students' initial exposure to the 'reality' of clinical medicine.

THE CLINICAL EXPERIENCE

Doctors' own reminiscences of their student days are full of vividly drawn accounts of their initial encounters with the mysteries of clinical medicine, and the awesome, theatrical, quirky or otherwise remarkable people who were responsible for their initiation. Those early, hesitant steps in clinical medicine mark a major turning-point in any doctor's individual, professional biography. It is part of the stock of personal mythology by which a doctor can trace out some of the salient features of his or her identity as a medical practitioner. Remembered with a mixture of fondness, pride and horror, these portraits of the past are familiar, and have been accurately lampooned by Ferris (1967): 'I well remember Sir Egbert telling me "always examine the patient in an easterly light".'

This is the very stuff of personal medical mythology. It also serves
to establish a collective, shared 'mythological charter'. For the
clinical tradition is central to the culture of medicine, and to the
transmission of that culture. 'Bedside medicine' and 'bedside teaching',
together with the knowledge that is produced and reproduced at the
bedside, is granted a privileged status in the clinical tradition.
Foucault (1973) has suggested that it is fundamental to the self
definition of 'modern' medicine. As Foucault describes it, 'the clinic'
is taken to provide the rationale for medicine's characteristic
empiricism, and the priority granted to firsthand, personal experience
and perception at the patient's bedside:

> Medicine has tended, since the eighteenth century, to recount
> its own history as if the patient's bedside had always been
> a place of constant, stable experience, in contrast to
> theories and systems which had been in perpetual change and
> masked beneath their speculation the purity of clinical
> evidence. (p.54)

The 'clinic', whose birth Foucault uncovers, was the distinctive
combination of new investigative technology, the reorganisation of
medical discourse, the rise of the great teaching hospitals and so on.
This conjuncture,he argues, produced a characteristic and revolutionary
mode of perception and understanding. Whereas previous theorising had
allowed for the natural history and classification of disease (often in
the most elaborate nosologies), the clinic was born when it became
permissible to treat the individual as a field of medical-clinical-
investigation: 'one could at last hold a scientifically structured
discourse about an individual'. The space by the patient's bedside thus
became a new locus of inquiry and research as well as treatment and
instruction.

In this 'clinical' space, the doctor's own direct scrutiny of the
patient became invested with a new significance. Under his gaze *(le
regard)* the superstructure of theory fell away to reveal a pure,
uncontaminated perception of the patient and his illness. Or such
became the mythological charter:

> Clinical experience...was soon taken as a simple,
> unconceptualized confrontation of a gaze and a face, or a
> glance and a silent body; a sort of contact prior to all
> discourse, free of all the burdens of language, by which
> two living individuals are 'trapped' in a common, but non
> reciprocal situation. (Foucault, 1973, p.xiv)

Foucault, of course, is arguing a very particular thesis concerning the
emergence of a novel system of thought and practice in revolutionary and
post-revolutionary France. In doing so he almost certainly over
emphasises the extent to which there was a radical break with the
medical past. The clinical gaze was granted a new and enhanced status,
but the clinical tradition and its mythology extends back, beyond
Foucault's moment of birth.

Any search for absolute origins is bound to fail, and it is in the
very nature of mythological charters that their remoter periods are
subject to change. Early generations are confused and compressed; the
relation of cult figures and heroes does not necessarily correspond to
the niceties of historical accuracy. But the figure of Boerhaave is

noteworthy in the development of eighteenth century clinical work. Foremost among the theorists and teachers at Leyden, Boerhaave's influence was profound and widespread. Appositely to this book, it was Boerhaave who provided the major influence on the early days of the medical school at Edinburgh. The medical school itself was established on the Continental model, and several of the early teachers were trained at Leyden, which was then the foremost centre of medical theory, practice and instruction (Comrie, 1932).

The practice of bedside teaching at Edinburgh, based on the Leyden model, was recognisably the predecessor of later approaches to clinical instruction, such as those Foucault describes:

> The Chief would go round the ward with his students and coming to a bed the Chief would stand at the top of the bed and the student would stand by the patient. The Chief would ask the student a question, the student would then speak to the patient, the patient would reply to the student, the student would shout at the top of his voice the answer to the assembled students and the Chief would hear the answer. (Eastwood, 1972)

In the eighteenth century, at medical schools like Leyden and Edinburgh, the clinical tradition was established. This 'old clinic' was a medicine of symptoms: there was little or no investigation of the patient's body for signs of pathology.

> The actual methods of teaching students were much the same in 1800 as they are today, with one great exception, the development of the technique of teaching due to that revolution in the technique of Medicine, the invention of the physical examination of the patient. This innovation demanded the introduction of methods of teaching the elicitation of physical signs, and the provision of those opportunities for practice and experience on which this interpretation and evaluation must be based. (Newman, 1957, p.30)

The clinical tradition established by Boerhaave and others in the eighteenth century, then, coupled with the new technology and emergent specialties of the nineteenth century, provides the basis for this mythological charter for medicine and its distinctive cultural reproduction. The emergence of the 'clinic' and its special status in the tradition of modern medicine has also been noted by Jamous and Peloille (1970). Their argument has many points of contact with Foucault's version. They describe how, during the early years of the last century, the roles of teacher, researcher and clinician became fused in the University hospitals in France. The hospital wards were the main research environment, as well as a locale for training and patient care. But as the century went on, this conjunction was threatened and fragmented. With the emergence of the laboratory based research (such as bacteriology), the clinician lost his monopoly over the production and use of medical knowledge. Within the medical profession, Jamous and Peloille argue, there emerged a struggle for supremacy between the clinicians and the non clinical scientists.

The detail of Jamous and Peloille's argument does not concern us here. They do, however, draw attention to the most important point. They document how hospital clinicians attempted to reassert their superiority

4

by means of appeals to their own pre-theoretical clinical experience.
By virtue of their clinical 'gaze' the clinicians laid claim to a
privileged perception. This arcane knowledge and experience was, it
was claimed, 'indeterminate', in contrast to the 'technical' rationality
of the 'scientific' disciplines. In their own discussion of actual
historical events, Jamous and Peloille are guilty of reifying their
notions of 'technicality' and 'indetermination' and of over simplifying
the historical relationships between competing definitions of medical
knowledge. Nonetheless, they are right to point out the centrality of
knowledge which is defined as 'indeterminate'. That is, knowledge
which practitioners believe is not susceptible to rational codification
and explicit statement. All crafts and occupations have such areas
(though the boundaries of technicality and indetermination will often
be disputed by members of occupational groups).

In the context of medicine, such 'indeterminate' knowledge has been
associated with the notion of 'clinical experience'. It has been
vouchsafed by the privilege of the 'clinical gaze'. This in turn, then,
has guaranteed the centrality of bedside teaching as the mode of
cultural transmission whereby such knowledge may be imparted. It
depends upon the novice, or apprentice, being exposed directly to the
signs and symptoms of illness. Despite the fragmentation of medical
knowledge and teaching, the growth of new specialities and the
increasing importance of science and technology, the 'clinic' and
bedside teaching have retained a central importance. Throughout the
changes in theory and practice of medical education, the clinical -
bedside teaching - has remained, in the essentials, unaltered. Its
justification remains that which Foucault and Jamous and Peloille
identify from earlier epochs - an appeal to direct, pre-theoretical
experience and the accumulation of personal, clinical experience.

If the clinic was born in the period described by Foucault, or in yet
earlier years, then it is re-born every day. It enjoys a daily
'renaissance' in the ward rounds of contemporary clinicians and their
students. In the training of medical students, their individual
biographies and the collective tradition of the medical profession flow
together. Here too are fused the components of 'theory' and 'practice'
of 'science' and 'practical experience' which are together taken to be
necessary for the production of competent members of the profession.

Clinical experience and the lessons of the bedside are, then, central
to the past and the present of the clinical culture. Such a distinctive
organisation of knowledge and perception gives rise to what Freidson
(1970) has described as the 'clinical mentality'. Freidson
distinguishes the medical practitioner, the clinician, from the theorist
or scientist. The clinician's primary orientation is towards action -
so much so that he or she may prefer to do something with very uncertain
chances of success over taking no action at all. The practitioner,
Freidson argues, 'believes in what he is doing'. That is, the clinician
is likely to display a personal commitment to his or her chosen course
of action. The practitioner is essentially a pragmatist, relying on
results rather than theory, and trusting in personal, firsthand
knowledge rather than on abstract principles or 'book knowledge'.

These components, all mutually interdependent, comprise a distinctive,
occupational culture, characterised by a particular orientation towards
knowledge and action. The clinical approach comes to induce in the

5

practitioner an ultimate trust in the evidence of his or her senses, and
the warrant of his or her personal knowledge (experience).   This
Freidson summarises as 'a rather thoroughgoing particularism, a kind of
ontological and epistemological individualism'.   It is the warrant for
individual action, and the competence of a practitioner may be judged
(e.g. by colleagues) by reference to the essentially biographical notion
of 'personal experience'.

   Freidson's remarks on the 'clinical mentality' are drawn in part from
Becker et al. (1961).   In their study of medical students at Kansas they
noted the importance of the 'experience perspective' in organising the
views of staff and students.   They summarise this perspective in this
way:

1.   It is important for a doctor to have had clinical
     experience.
2.   School activities are good insofar as they give students
     the opportunity to acquire clinical experience or give
     them access to the clinical experience of their teachers;
     they are bad when they furnish neither of these things.
3.   A student is making real progress towards his goal of
     preparing for practise when he can demonstrate to himself
     and others that he has absorbed some lessons from
     clinical experience;   conversely, he has cause to be
     worried over his own abilities when he fails to absorb
     such lessons.   (p.242)

   Although it is not the only available criterion, the notion of
'clinical experience' is often used as a touchstone in the evaluation of
some course of action, or in choosing between competing approaches.   As
Becker et al. go on to comment, 'actual experience in dealing with
patients and disease' is often used in contrast to 'theoretical' and
'scientific' knowledge:

     ...even though it substitutes for scientifically verified
     knowledge, it can be used to legitimate a choice of
     procedures for a patient's treatment and can even be used
     to rule out use of some procedures that have been
     scientifically established.   (p.225)

In this context, 'scientifically established' should not be understood
in any absolute sense.   What is at issue is what passes for up to date,
validated scientific procedure - incorporated in research papers,
learned journals, textbooks and so on.   'Scientific' knowledge and
'personal experience' are equally social in their definition, but the
warrants claimed for them are different.

   The clinical culture is predicated therefore on the personal
accumulation of clinical experience, and such a stock of knowledge is an
essential component of any practitioner's competence.   It is acquired in
large measure at the patient's bedside - that personal and perceptual
space encompassed by the clinical gaze.

   Historically speaking the 'apprenticeship' model of medical training
has become somewhat attenuated.   The attachment of a young novice
doctor to the 'firm' of a mentor no longer plays the part it once did,
and is but one of a wide range of educational experiences the medical
student is exposed to.   Similarly, the student's actual responsibility

for the day to day care of the patient has been postponed. The student is no longer, as Flexner (1925) described, 'part of the functioning machine'. Junior medical students in their early days of clinical medicine or surgery are much less frequently expected to undertake the routine and menial tasks once expected of a 'clerk' or 'dresser'.

Nonetheless, the underlying mode of teaching and learning retains core features of 'apprenticeship'. Though junior students do not play an important part in the daily work of the ward, they still gain their clinical understanding through exposure to the clinical world of the hospital. Students are expected to acquire their expertise, and to accumulate their store of experience, largely from the example of their clinical teachers. They learn by example: by observing at the bedside, in the clinic, from the gallery or on the floor of the operating theatre. They acquire their competence through supervised practical work, in the 'real-life' context of medical practice. Even though their diagnoses and opinions are not actually implemented and do not normally affect the management of patients, students are called upon to examine, diagnose and prescribe treatment as if they were indeed responsible for the patients they encounter. Although they are not usually entrusted with work of real importance, junior students learn 'on the job'.

In the transmission of the clinical culture, its enactment in 'bedside teaching' is of fundamental importance. But despite its centrality to medical education and its mythological significance, bedside teaching has remained almost entirely neglected as a topic of sociological research.

THE INVISIBLE CLINIC

Medical students are often used as a benchmark in the literature on professional socialisation, as well as in the sociology of medicine. The place of medical education has been secured in the sociological literature by two classic studies. The first was based upon the teaching programme at Cornell, and was undertaken by members of the Columbia University Bureau of Applied Social Research (Merton et al., 1957). The second, a study of Kansas University medical school was done by members of a research group in sociology at the University of Chicago (Becker et al., 1961). The contrasting portrayals of medical education and student life offered by these two studies have become reference points in the literature on professional socialisation. For lack of comparable research in this country, commentators have all too often been content to assimilate British experience to one or other of the American examples.

Arguably, the undoubted quality and importance of the two 'classics' has had an inhibiting effect on subsequent researchers, both in Britain and elsewhere. There has been, I suspect, a willingness on the part of many British sociologists to believe that medical education has been 'done', and to rely almost exclusively on the American sources. Elsewhere, notably in the United States, subsequent research has been undertaken. But the inhibitory effect of the early studies is apparent nonetheless. There is a tendency for later research almost obsessively to recapitulate the problems and perspectives laid down by the Columbia and Chicago studies (Atkinson, forthcoming). Admittedly those themes nature of 'professions' and 'professional socialisation', which in turn reflect divergences in sociological theory and method in general. It is not my intention to review this debate in any detail, but a brief summary is unavoidable.

While they have been fascinated by 'the professions' for many years, sociologists have, while claiming to demystify them, been mystified in their turn (cf. Roth, 1974). Sociological observers of the professions have repeatedly found themselves entangled in a web of definitional problems. Indeed, the very meaning of the term 'profession' and 'professional' have proved a stumbling block, and their value as sociological concepts has been much contested.

In simple terms one can identify two competing approaches: one which seeks to identify 'professions' as distinctive, special sorts of occupations, and one which denies any inherent qualities which might set them apart. The first approach takes as a dominant theme the identification of the *differentia specifica* of the professions. In some of their characteristic forms such approaches are referred to as 'trait' theories. The task of delineating a distinctive category of 'professions' has proved troublesome. Many of the proposed lists have proved incompatible; while all or some of the traits appear to apply to so-called professions, they apply also to occupations not so designated; often it is far from clear where the traits are derived from; many of the characteristics appear to have been incorporated from the occupations' public self presentation and 'bootlegged' into the sociologists' definitions.

The second approach avoids such pitfalls. It derives in large measure from the work of Everett Hughes (1958). The crucial question, it is maintained, is not 'what is a profession?', but rather 'when do people begin to apply this label to themselves?' In other words, 'profession' and 'professional' are self designations or claims made for and by particular occupational groups. There is, according to this view, nothing inherent in the work or training, nor in the personnel, which denotes 'professions' as a particular class of occupation.

The first approach, associated with functionalist theorising, coloured the research of the Columbia group, and their account of medical education. The latter, distinctively interactionist perspective, underlies the work of the Chicago school.

Merton and his collaborators have in mind a distinctive set of roles and values as the *terminus ad quem* of training: medical students are

> engaged in learning the professional role of the physician
> by so combining its component knowledge and skills,
> attitudes and values, as to be motivated and able to
> perform their role in a professionally and socially
> acceptable fashion. (p.41)

In this view the distinctive knowledge, attitudes and values of the fully fledged professional are seen as being laid down during the initial training period.

Becker and his colleagues, on the other hand, stress the immediate, day to day experience of medical school life, and play down the relationship between basic education and future performance as a competent practitioner. Rather than assuming the assimilation of a repertoire of roles and values, the Chicago researchers concentrate on how students survive and they get through medical school.

The two approaches can be seen as attempts, more or less successful, to answer two different questions. The Columbia study asks, 'How do people become doctors?' The emphasis of the Chicago study is rather focused on 'learning the ropes'; initiates are faced with immediate, practical problems of 'getting by' in novel situations and must find ways of coping. Miller (1970, p.118) summarises this approach succinctly:

> Newcomers in any social situation go through an initial process
> of learning the ropes: finding out who the other people in
> that situation are, where they are located, what they do, what
> they expect the newcomer to do, and how they want him to do it.
> We seldom dignify this process by calling it learning.

Yet it is precisely this aspect of 'learning' that is seized on by Becker and his co-workers.

In line with these differing perspectives, too, the two studies portray student life in very different terms - aptly caught in their respective titles. The 'student physician' is described as a junior partner in the training process, who is sponsored toward full membership of the profession by his teachers. The 'boy in white' is seen as occupying a much more lowly position, and enjoying very different relationships with medical school staff. There is a strong social barrier between the staff and students and a divergence between their respective preoccupations and interests. Each study describes a 'student culture', but ascribes very different characteristics to them. The Columbia research describes student culture as comprising a 'little society' in which the professional norms of the faculty are reflected and reinforced. At Kansas, the student culture appears almost to be an 'underground resistance movement', in which students unite against a hostile and threatening environment.

These two positions, to a considerable extent, have provided taken for granted reference points, either in terms of guiding subsequent work, or inhibiting more original approaches (Atkinson, forthcoming). But they do not represent the only possible perspectives. Neither their subject matter nor their approaches to medical education are exhaustive. There have been major *lacunae* in their coverage (and in subsequently published research projects). In particular both the Columbia study and the Chicago-school research at Kansas neglected the topic of clinical teaching. Merton and his colleagues focus on students' attitudes towards medicine and types of patients, but remain silent on the nature of the student-patient encounter. Likewise, Becker and his co-authors remark on students' attitudes; but 'Students and Patients' is given only brief attention, and 'Student-Patient Interaction' occupies a bare two pages of what is a lengthy monograph. More recent studies of medical education have also tended to gloss over the particular topic of clinical, bedside instruction.

Perhaps the most disappointing of all these omissions is that of the Chicago school. The authors note that 'The student spends much of his time in the clinical years interacting with patients', they offer only a brief idealised description of the student-patient encounter:

The third year student typically meets his patients when they are hospitalised for diagnosis and treatment. He comes into contact with them repeatedly during their hospital stay. He performs a complete examination upon the patient's arrival in the hospital. He presents the patient to the staff and other students during the rounds, describing the case in detail, demonstrating outstanding clinical findings, and suggesting a diagnosis and plan of treatment. He checks daily on the patient's progress, quizzing and re-examining the patient frequently. He enters into a casual but continuing relationship with the patient. The major problem patients present for the student on the hospital wards, then, is to maintain this continuing relationship in such a fashion as to be able to get the necessary information he is assigned. (p.315)

In this highly compressed account, then, Becker and his colleagues gloss over a wide range of skills, problems and social encounters: students must engage in purposeful talk with patients, perform examinations, formulate histories and generate diagnoses. Students must generate displays of ability, under the scrutiny of their clinical teachers, and present a 'front' of competence. In the context of such encounters, and through social accomplishments, medical knowledge is transmitted in a dramatic fashion. Yet all this has remained strangely neglected.

Bedside teaching has remained largely unexamined from within medicine. While medical school members have themselves engaged vigorously in research and innovation, they have tended to concentrate on such topics as methods of selection and assessment, career choice, psychological assessment and so on. One author (Crooks, 1974) has been moved to describe the topic of bedside clinical instruction as 'taboo'.

To some extent the state of research reflects dominant interests on the part of both sociological observers, and medical educators. But the neglect of bedside teaching may go rather deeper than that. It may lie in the nature of the enterprise itself and its taken for granted legitimacy, in that it apparently depends on the students' direct exposure to the 'reality' of medical work. Such firsthand experience may appear to need no further elaboration or justification. It can appear so 'obvious' and 'natural' that direct observation and investigation in turn appear unnecessary. Just as bedside work provides a traditional justification for the distinctive clinical culture, so it has a self-justificatory aim in its day to day accomplishment.

Bedside teaching may also have remained relatively invisible for another reason. Crooks' description of clinical instruction as 'taboo' seems particularly apt. There is more than a hint that bedside experience is regarded as the most 'sacred' of the mysteries which only the initiated may be party to. Exposure to this world constitutes a core of the extended *rite de passage* of the medical student.

Although there has been a considerable amount of curricular innovation in British medical schools in recent years, the centrality of clinical instruction in the major hospital subjects (primarily medicine and surgery) has remained. Introductory courses in clinical method tend to be focused on the 'classical' concerns of history taking, physical

examination and diagnostic inference on the wards of the teaching
hospital. The 'clinic' remains self evidently at the heart of the
'clinical', and the 'clinic' at the heart of medical training.

2 Entering the Clinical World

The Royal Infirmary - the main teaching hospital at Edinburgh - stands
next to the quadrangle of the Faculty of Medicine, which contains the
laboratories and lecture theatres, library etc. The two are separated
by a tree lined walk which leads into the Meadows, a large park.
Student tradition has it that it is a matter of some moment whether, on
arriving first thing in the morning, one turns east into the preclinical building, or west, into the Infirmary. The physical proximity
of the two sets of buildings and their separation mirrors the divide
between the two main phases of the undergraduate curriculum, and a
decisive break in students' careers. The majority of students regard
the transition from 'preclinical' to 'clinical' work as a particularly
critical status passage in the course of their training.   The
undergraduate curriculum at Edinburgh follows the traditional pattern
in dividing the course into these two major segments - the preclinical
and the clinical. Students spend two or three years in the preclinical
phase, depending on their entry qualifications. Students begin their
clinical work in the fourth year of the course overall.

The fourth year student's day begins with a lecture in a course on
'the nature of disease'. In the early weeks of the year, these lectures
provide an 'introduction to clinical medicine', and include lectures on
such general topics as: 'the approach to the patient': 'history-taking -
the present complaint'; 'factors in the history-previous, environmental
and genetic'; 'observation of the patient'. From then on the lecture
course proceeds system by system, with talks from members of staff from
various clinical and non clinical departments. This course of formal
lectures on clinical topics is an attempt to provide a unifying element
in an otherwise fragmentary clinical component.

After their lecture the students make their way to various clinical
attachments in the teaching hospitals. The fourth year introductory
teaching takes place in five of the hospitals associated with the
university - the Royal Infirmary, the Western General, the Eastern
General, the Northern General and the Leith Hospitals. During the first
term of the year the fourth year students are all attached to medical
units. In the second and third terms they are attached to a surgical
unit and a second unit in medicine.

The groups in which the students are attached to medical and surgical
units are known as 'cliniques', a term redolent of Edinburgh's close
historical associations with the tradition of European medicine. In the
first term, these groups (in medicine) contain about a dozen students.
Later in the year the groups are rather smaller.

These cliniques provide the students with a closely defined group of
peers with whom they interact, with whom they work, and with whom they
share their everyday experiences. Even though not all members of a
clinique are close or even friendly before the group is formed at the
start of a term, they become acquainted through sharing their clinical
work. In these groups students negotiate their common views of shared

problems, or debate their differences of opinion. On the wards, between teaching periods, in hospital canteens, waiting in corridors, on the coach between the university and an outlying hospital, the members of a clinique can chatter and reflect together on the teaching they are receiving, the patients they have seen, the characteristics of the clinicians and so on.

The general pattern of a clinical unit comprises male and female wards, a teaching room, the normal procedure rooms, doctors' and nurses' rooms and so on. Each clinical unit is staffed by a small number of consultants, plus their 'firms' of registrars and housemen. The majority of such units are staffed by NHS clinicians, who hold honorary university appointments, or part time teaching appointments. Some are university based units: the staff hold positions as professors, senior lecturers and lecturers, and have honorary appointments as consultants and registrars. These 'professorial' units tend to have larger complements of staff than their NHS counterparts.

One consultant described the arrangement of units as being 'like a series of cottage hospitals', referring to the degree of autonomy enjoyed by each. Each group of doctors takes the responsibility for arranging the teaching of the fourth year students, and for arranging this to fit in with their other work of patient care, research and administration. The particular staffing arrangements and practicalities of day to day organisation mean that the precise organisation and content of the teaching vary considerably from attachment to attachment. But there are common types of teaching that are generally found from unit to unit. These are the major types of clinical instruction and clinical encounter which are recognised and distinguished by staff and students themselves.

Bedside teaching. I have already presented a sketch of such teaching, and it is familiar. A doctor takes a group of students into the ward and teaches at a patient's bedside. The clinician may spend all of the time with just one patient, or conduct a 'round', teaching on a number of patients in succession. Such teaching provides occasion for students to learn and practise the techniques of history-taking and physical examination. Physicians and surgeons themselves can demonstrate such skills to the students. An individual patient and his or her problems may serve as a starting point for a more general discussion of pathology, clinical method, management and so on.

Tutorials. Doctors may conduct small group teaching sessions of a more 'theoretical' nature, without direct recourse to the patients on the wards. These take place in the teaching rooms. On some units there are regular series of tutorials, on others they take place on an *ad hoc* basis. The teaching room may also be used for the discussion of points of interest that arise at the bedside and which the teaching clinician wishes to develop further; the room is often resorted to in order to avoid a discussion of potentially worrying or distressing features of a case within earshot of the patient.

'Waiting nights'. The individual hospital units receive emergency admissions on a rota basis. On their 'receiving' or 'waiting' nights, fourth year students attached to a unit are expected to attend for at least part of the evening. Usually the students come in small numbers, members of the clinique taking it in turns to come in in twos and

threes. On waiting nights the students are able to see patients who are admitted to the hospital in the acute phases of various conditions (such as myocardical infarctions in medicine, acute abdomens in surgery). Students have the chance to accompany doctors when they admit patients, see them take an initial history and examine the patient. They can be present when early differential diagnoses are formulated by the admitting doctor and management initiated. On surgical attachments waiting nights provide opportunities for students to go into theatre, and observe operations taking place. From time to time the students may even have the chance to assist in the operating theatre, in a humble fashion, by holding a retractor.

Ward Meetings. These occasions are not specifically designed as teaching occasions, but are, in a way, educational for all those concerned. Staff and students come together to discuss cases that they have on the wards. Cases are presented by senior students or members of staff, or someone may be asked to give a brief presentation on a specific topic of general interest; rarely a fourth year student may be asked to work up a patient for presentation. One of the pathologists may come to the meeting and discuss in detail the findings of biopsies, the results of post mortem examinations and so on. By and large the fourth year students take little active part in these meetings, though the doctor will pause to explain points of interest to them, ask them questions, check whether they understand the proceedings and so on.

Clerking. As well as seeing patients with clinical teachers in small groups, students may also be given the task of seeing patients individually. This activity, usually referred to as 'clerking' a patient, is designed to allow students to take a full history and perform a full physical examination on a patient. When done thoroughly this takes the student a number of hours, possibly spread over a number of days, and on some days of the week a period of time is set aside (on some units) for students to get this work done on one or more patients. Members of a clinique may thus have patients allocated to them on a weekly basis - a list of students and 'their' patients is posted at the beginning of the week. On completion of the history and examination the students are usually required to write up the case notes and to formulate a differential diagnosis, as if they were responsible for the admission of the patient. The case notes are read and commented on by a staff member. From time to time a period may be set aside for the clinique members to go over the notes and findings together, and to present cases to each other.

The bedside teaching and clerking that are discussed here cannot be taken as 'typical' of all British medical education in all its details. There has always been something of a difference in emphasis between the Scottish medical schools and their English counterparts (especially the London schools). In England the tendency has been to use the 'apprenticeship' system, with the student 'walking the wards', while in Scotland there has been an emphasis on small group teaching at the bedside. At Edinburgh students do not routinely become involved with the day to day care of individual patients. The form of 'clerking' that they do is therefore an important way in which such involvement can be approximated on the wards.

Since the students do not have responsibility for the care of patients, the main focus of the fourth year is a grounding for the students in basic clinical method. Emphasis is placed on students' acquisition of methods and routines of clinical inquiry. There is less emphasis placed upon the management of patients and the practicalities of diagnostic or therapeutic work.

In addition to the general teaching arrangements already referred to, there is a range of other opportunities available to students. They may be able to attend post mortem examinations. At least one of the hospitals announced that such an event was taking place with a discrete notice *Sectio Hodie*. When students see the notice they are supposed to inform the clinician on their unit; if the dead person was one of their patients, and if it is thought 'interesting' or 'valuable', then the clinique attend the post mortem.

At times students attend out patient clinics. They 'sit in' on consultations between the doctor and the succession of patients whom he sees. The students may also be called upon to question or examine the patient themselves. There are, too, clinical lectures once a week in the Royal Infirmary for students in cliniques there. One of the consultants addresses the students in a lecture theatre. He may bring one or more of his own patients along from the wards in order to illustrate the them of the lecture, the patients being wheeled in in their beds. Attendance at these lectures is rather patchy and many students 'skive off'. (They do feel constrained to attend the lecture if it is being delivered by a consultant from their own wards, lest their absence be noted and held against them). Students often go along to these clinical lectures in order to 'have a look' at the various consultants, rather than seeing them as a major part of their clinical work. There is more than a hint of a theatrical display, in which the students learn more about the doctors' styles of performance than clinical medicine.

One of the most dramatic and absorbing experiences for students in the fourth year is their early introduction to surgery. Although they do not necessarily take active part in the actual performance of operations, the students get an opportunity to observe the work of the surgeons in the operating theatre. The theatres are equipped with galleries from which clinique members can watch what is going on. The surgeons can address remarks to the students, or provide a running commentary on the operation they are performing. Surgeons can stop and point out structures to the students, or quiz them on aspects of anatomy that they should know. Students may also observe from the floor of an operating theatre. It is, in fact, rather hard to see very much of what is going on during many operations. The small huddle of surgeons, anaesthetist and nurses block off a clear view of the action. The students often find themselves looking at the backs and bent heads of the operating team.

Rather like the first days in the anatomy dissecting rooms, a student's first operation may be seen as major landmarks in a student's growing repository of experiences. Like the introduction to anatomy, too, this experience is sometimes regarded with slight misgivings. But the novelty soon wears off, and it becomes one of the taken for granted things which students come to accept. Nonetheless, visits to the operating theatres do provide the students with valued opportunities for firsthand observation of the 'real' work of hospital surgery.

The precise arrangements for clinical work vary from unit to unit, but the general pattern is similar across them all. For students, the differences between cliniques are important, but the transition to clinical work is the most fundamental qualitative change that they recognise. While they have grumbles about aspects of their clinical work, the students are all agreed that it is preferable to the preclinical segment of the course. As one student expressed it:

> This year, the actual stuff isn't easier, but it's more
> interesting and it's easier to remember. When you see a
> patient with the disease process it's easier to remember;
> also it's easier to learn when you're taught in small
> groups....

Interest in the work of the clinical years is a recurrent theme in students' views of their time on the wards. One of the women students went so far as to say that she was now 'looking forward to Monday mornings' - something that certainly had not been true during the earlier part of the course. For her things had been getting progressively better: the second year was 'shocking', the third year 'better', and as for the fourth year, she was actually 'enjoying it': it was

> ...much more interesting than preclinical....There's
> much less awful swotting. Because it's interesting
> I think you pick it up more easily.

For the students, the 'interest' lay primarily in the perceived 'reality' and 'relevance' of their clinical studies, as opposed to the 'academic' nature of the preclinical years. Dealing with patients is seen not only as inherently more interesting and absorbing, but also helps to put into perspective the material that has been (or should have been) assimilated in the second and third years. This is attributed to

> The fact that you talk to patients, have actual contact
> with them, and the fact that you can see why you studied
> the stuff in the other three years makes it all worthwhile.

And as another student put it:

> It's nice to have some contact with patients....You learn
> more by application this year than by rote, like we did
> last year.

Indeed students would explain that sometimes they only really learned or understood some aspect of the preclinical syllabus when they began to encounter it in a clinical context. Anatomy and physiology particularly came into their own during the basic clinical training of the fourth year. In surgery, for instance, I often observed the surgeons 'revising' anatomy which they at least seemed to think the students should have known. Neuroanatomy and the anatomy of the peripheral vascular system, which were treated as important on at least some surgical units, were topics which students had to re-learn in the context of actual surgical problems and procedures.

It is not hard, of course, to see how the various scientific 'facts' could be learned more readily in the clinical context. Individual patients provide the most memorable of 'audio-visual aids' in the

demonstration of illness. They furnish vivid exemplification, a
dramatic enactment of medical concerns. On the basis of my own period
of research, I can vouch for the memorability of clinical presentations.
The individual patients I saw with the students remain fresh in my mind.
For the students, their first patient with distinctive signs and
symptoms of a particular disease remains fresh in the memory, in a way
which the de-contextualised 'facts' of a textbook or the lecture theatre
do not.

The fourth year students, then, welcome the move into the clinical
phase as a shift towards the 'real' work of medicine, and away from the
'academic', 'theoretical' and 'scientific' aspects of their course.
Apart from periods of vacation work for some of them, the transfer marks
the students' first sustained contact with practising doctors and their
patients in the milieu of 'real' medical work.

The majority of students do not envisage entering non clinical medical
work, such as research, epidemiology or public health. They see their
eventual career involving direct contact with patients, either on
hospital wards and clinics, or in general practice. While many do not
have a precise speciality in mind, they are still committed to a future
in clinical work of some sort. It is, therefore, hardly surprising that
they should see the preclinical sciences as little better than something
of a 'chore', a major hurdle to be negotiated before the 'real' work of
medicine as such.

The authors of the Royal Commission on Medical Education (1968) noted
that the division into preclinical and clinical stages can induce
malaise among students during the early years of such a course, as well
as being a potential source of dissatisfaction on the part of members of
teaching staff in medical schools:

> The two stages are often thought to be too sharply divided and
> from the student's viewpoint the division is exaggerated by
> the Second Professional Examination...clinicians argue that
> not enough weight is given to clinical aspects of the medical
> sciences, while teachers of the preclinical subjects claim
> with equal force that their task is to give a solid grounding
> in science, leaving its clinical application until later.
> Many students allege that the preclinical subjects as taught
> to them appear to have so little relevance to practical
> medicine that they find the early part of their course
> discouraging and their interest is aroused only when they
> reach the clinical stage. (p.87)

The fourth year students at Edinburgh certainly treat the division as a
major one, and tended to look back on the preclinical years as drudgery.
The overall course is long, and students are eager to complete it as
rapidly as possible. The preparation for the 'Second MB' examination is
looked back on by fourth years as a time of considerable emotional
stress and intellectual effort. In comparison, their introduction to
clinical work seemed very easy and relaxed, apparently requiring much
less sustained effort and concentration. As one of the girls put it,
'The third year was terrible...this year is much easier', and, as
another said, 'You can go at a slower pace'.

The students' experience of work in the medical school is therefore paradoxical. They find themselves working heavily on matters which they do not find absorbing, or relevant to their future career; they feel less heavily committed when they come on to work which seems more central to their medical training. Ellis (1975) has remarked that in comparison with the 'tread-mill' for much of the undergraduate years, 'the long clinical course all too easily lacks any sense of urgency'.

The status passage from the preclinical years is therefore welcomed by the students on two counts. Their new work is both 'easier', and more gripping. The very organisation of the formal curriculum tends to imply that the preclinical years are to be thought of as preparation for more important work. The whole undergraduate curriculum appears to follow a simple logic - from the 'pure theory' of the basic sciences to pure 'practical experience'. The first clinical year therefore conveys the impression of a significant staging post in the sequence from theory to practice.

The clinicians themselves tend to reinforce this perception. They too stress a qualitative difference between the two phases. Rather than continuity between the preclinical and clinical aspects, they tend to emphasise the fact that the students are 'starting again'. For instance, during the first week of my fieldwork one of the younger consultants on the medical unit I was observing told the clinique, 'You are in the delicate position of forgetting your physiology and learning medicine'.

> The students from various cliniques - about thirty of them -
> were taken for a demonstration of X-ray techniques. They all
> sat round and were invited to comment on a number of X-ray
> pictures that were put up at the front of the class, and to
> compare them with a 'normal' film which was also displayed.
> One girl made a suggestion that was, I gathered, way off
> target. Dr Mason (one of the consultant physicians)
> commented to the radiologist, "They're allowed to say
> anything, you know; they don't know any medicine yet".

Just as the students find they need to re-learn their preclinical subjects in the context of bedside work, so the clinicians emphasise this to the students. In medicine, for instance, I noted that neurology was often described as little more than an applied knowledge of the underlying anatomy, and usually coupled with criticism of the students' apparent ignorance of that anatomy. Similarly, the surgeons would often be at pains to rehearse basic anatomy while discussing operative techniques, discussing the findings of a particular case, looking at X-rays and so on.

As I shall go on to discuss in greater detail later, the clinicians would lay stress on 'clinical' knowledge, contrasting it with both the theories of text books, and the teachings of non clinical scientists, to the detriment of the latter. For instance, a junior physician was teaching the students in a 'tutorial', and asked the students for the cause of a particular condition:

St: Myocarditis....

Dr: (derisively) Yah!

St: Well, that's the pathological description that's
     given for it.

Dr: Pathology's finished. We're on clinical work here;
           pathology's waffle, just cover-up stuff.

Similarly, I noted the following exchange between a consultant surgeon
and the members of a clinique:

Dr: So there's an example of course of a goitre in a
           patient of thirty six - of long standing, eighteen
           years. So you are in a little difficulty if it
           isn't nodular. You've finished with thyroid
           pathology?

St: Yes.

Dr: So what is it?

St: If it isn't nodular, it might be adenoma of the
           thyroid.

Dr: Hmm...I sometimes think that pathologists have a
           distorted view of thyroid pathology. By adenoma
           I suppose you mean a simple tumour?

St: Yes.

Dr: Simple tumours of the thyroid are very rare....

The consultant then went on to ask the students about the age of the
onset of goitre.

St: Onset of puberty.

Dr: You're quite right that the text books talk of
           adolescent goitre, but....

and he went on to explain that the students should not rely on what the
text books said on the matter.

In this particular exchange, the surgeon managed to contrast his own
clinical approach both with the niceties of pathologists' theorising,
and the received wisdom enshrined in text books. Such contrasts were
by no means uncommon, and they provide a recurrent reinforcement of the
primacy of clinical knowledge over 'theory'. Often such presentation
of knowledge stresses that the clinical is more down to earth, less
concerned with pettifogging detail and exceptional cases. The
clinician portrays himself as a pragmatist. Not, that is, that the
clinician promotes a view of his knowledge as crude or unsophisticated;
his is the subtlety of experience grounded in painstakingly accumulated
knowledge of the 'real world', not based on the theoretician's
theoretical or experimental excursions.

In a number of ways, then, the students who enter their first
clinical year feel that they have embarked on a novel and valuable
segment of their careers. Many of them for the first time feel
themselves gripped and absorbed by the world of 'real' medicine that
they now encounter. One girl described her experience of the first
term of clinical medicine as 'intoxicating', and many of her classmates
too found it heady stuff.

This subjective experience of transition reflects what Davis (1968)
has called the process of 'doctrinal conversion'. Davis seeks to
capture 'those feeling states, inner turning points and experiential
markings which, from the perspective of the subject, impart a

characteristic tone, meaning and quality to his status passage'. Davis draws on the very apt metaphor coined by Hughes (1958, p.119):

> One might say that the learning of the medical role consists of a separation, almost an alienation of the student from the lay medical world; a passing through the mirror so that one looks out at the world from behind it, and sees things as in mirror writing.

In all the more 'esoteric occupations', Hughes suggests, one finds this sense of seeing the world 'in reverse'. During the period of training and initiation, two cultures - the 'lay' and the 'professional' - interact. Hughes remarks that such interaction goes on throughout an individual's life.

> ...but it seems to be more lively - more exciting and uncomfortable, more self-conscious and yet perhaps more deeply unconscious - in the period of learning and initiation. (p.119)

In the 'professions', as Hughes observes, the process of 'passing through the mirror' is most apparent. The sense of 'difference', the sense of separation between the practitioner and the layman is most marked. Most studies of professional 'socialisation' have tended to concentrate on how the novice comes to take on the appropriate perspectives and understandings, behaviour and values which characterise their newly-gained occupational culture.

Important though such concerns are, there has been a tendency to ignore or gloss over one crucial aspect of such occupational cultures - and because of the process of 'doctrinal conversion'. While observers puzzle over the mysterious process whereby, say, medical students become doctors, they are in danger of overlooking one rather important component - that in the course of their years in medical school they learn medicine! Stated thus the observation seems quite absurdly trivial. But it is the case that what makes for the 'esoteric' nature of such occupations as medicine lies (in great measure) in the expertise which is their stock in trade. Irrespective of the actual, ultimate value of the occupation's accumulated wisdom, the knowledge and skills employed by practitioners is the cornerstone of their collective licence and mandate (cf. Hughes 1958). The acquisition of such competence underlies, too, the individual's subjective experience of doctrinal conversion. The medical student, after all, is not only taking on board values, attitudes and perspectives; he or she is engaged in the rapid - at times almost frenzied - accumulation of medical knowledge.

In the course of their training, students of 'the professions' in particular achieve some mastery over complex and powerful systems of explanation and understanding. They are powerful in the sense that they encompass many areas of personal and public concern, providing frameworks for interpretation and intervention in many aspects of everyday life. They are, of course, 'powerful' too in the sense that they confer power, influence and prestige on those who manipulate them.

It is not surprising, therefore, that initiates should become fascinated by these realms of discourse and understanding. It has been noted in a number of different contexts that the vocabularies of expertise become incorporated into trainees' everday accounts of themselves and others. Bucher and Stelling (1977, p.103), for instance, describe how one group of residents in psychiatry acquired and began to use their technical vocabulary to describe the supervisory process while talking about their relationships with superiors: 'There was an enormously detailed, elaborated description of each supervisor in terms of his character structure and the nature of his interaction and contribution to the supervision'.

In part, the use of such technical vocabularies in ordering experience can be seen as an element in 'role-playing' or 'role simulation'. Davis (1968), for instance, identifies simulation as a stage in the process of conversion, describing a 'genre of highly self-conscious, manipulative behaviour of students which aims at constructing institutionally valued performances of a particular role'. Students thus enact a somewhat uncertain version of what they take to be appropriate professional activity. This view, which is echoed by Olesen and Whittaker (1968) follows a fairly familiar dramaturgical view of the student actor, involved in 'psyching out' their teachers and presenting a 'front', or favourable self-presentation.

Undoubtedly there is a good deal in this. Students do find themselves, more or less self-consciously, 'playing' at being doctors or nurses without feeling that they are really comfortable and at home in such activity. They subjectively experience themselves as occupying a 'liminal' position, neither fully competent experts nor still laymen. Yet to attribute students' use of their newly found, embryonic expertise simply to such manipulative role playing misses much of the students' experience.

In particular, the seductive appeal of much expert knowledge escapes such a perspective. As I have already indicated, it is part of the appeal of many bodies of esoteric knowledge that they furnish frames of reference which, apparently, account for many facets of human behaviour. They have connotations of revelation: they may offer insight into human motives, actions, problems and sufferings. The daily doings of one's fellows are a constant source of fascination, and the 'expert' is afforded privileged access to the private lives of others, while enjoying the licence to intervene in them. In the case of medicine, students gain firsthand experience of the troubles of a very varied range of people, while at the same time learning how to intervene in order to cure or alleviate them.

It is, therefore, small wonder that the novice, in the process of gaining competence in manipulating his or her developing expertise, should find them, quite literally, absorbing. Elsewhere, I have written, in a fairly lighthearted way, of the well known phenomenon of 'medical students' disease' - that is, the hypochondria to which medical students are prone. It has been suggested that this is largely the outcome of heightened stress and anxiety on the students' part, in the face of extreme academic pressure. While this may play a part, I would prefer to suggest that all we need to postulate to account for students' hypochondria is not heightened anxiety, but a heightened awareness of the clinical. Students become more or less adept at handling a complex symbolic domain in which disease categories and diagnostic inference figure pre-eminently. It should therefore come as little surprise that clinical understanding should come to occupy a dominant position in students' repertoire of conceptual schemes. Certainly the fourth year students at Edinburgh applied candidate diagnoses to themselves as well as to others - to their teachers, at times, as well as to their patients. That they did so simply reflects the centrality of the 'clinical' to the everyday experience of the student in his or her first clinical year.

It may be reasonable to account for such occasions as 'playful'. Certainly students 'play' with their stethoscopes, and with their tendon hammers. I often observed students engrossed in bashing their own knees with their hammers, producing repeated knee-jerks. But in describing it as 'play' we should not assume that we are dealing with self-conscious, manipulative action: to do so overlooks the fact that in 'play' we become absorbed, given over entirely to the activity in hand. The student who was 'intoxicated' with clinical work was describing something more totally gripping than simple simulation.

The fourth year students, in their initial encounters with clinical medicine, I am suggesting, become absorbed, seduced almost, by the clinical gaze. This particular doctrinal conversion occurs in the context of the teaching hospital, where the clinic is enacted, wherein the students are initiated into the mysteries of their craft. For students and staff alike, the importance of clinical, bedside teaching is self evident. Its legitimacy is guaranteed by virtue of the students' exposure to, and immersion in, the 'real world' of everyday life on the wards. In contrast with the abstract, academic worlds of the lecture theatre and the laboratory, on the hospital wards the students can engage directly with the very stuff of medicine. Its authenticity is thus self justifying. The rest of this book will be largely devoted to examining the nature of this clinical 'reality' and its 'authenticity'. My argument will be that this 'reality' is artfully stage managed and constructed in such a way as to reproduce particular versions of medical work and a particular form of medical culture.

3 Counting Experience and Organizing Careers

JUDGING CLINIQUES

In the course of their first clinical year the students have an interest in the accumulation of 'clinical experience', and in the organisation of their student careers. For most of them this is the first time when they exercise choice in charting a personal course through the medical school. For each of the three terms of the year students are asked to state their preference as to which clinique they should like to attend. Although it does not guarantee attachment to a particular unit, a student's choice does significantly affect the chances of a placement, and hence the nature of the clinical experience he or she amasses.

Each of the clinical units available in medicine and surgery enjoys a high degree of autonomy with regard to the provision made for undergraduate teaching. Each clinical unit develops its own arrangements, which reflect the clinical and educational commitments of the staff members involved. Each unit can, in theory at least, offer the student a unique educational experience. It is, therefore, an important part of the 'art and practice of studentmanship' (Olesen and Whittaker, 1968) that students should attempt to acquire and use information which they believe to be relevant to their choices between the various medical and surgical cliniques. On the basis of such information, they need to plan an undergraduate career which best satisfies their personal plans.

This interest is a major preoccupation of the local 'student culture'. Becker and Geer (1960) describe such culture in this way:

> This culture grows around those problems shared by all
> students in the school, problems related to their manifest
> identities as students: the immediate necessity of
> mastering a vast amount of factual material, the more
> distant threat of failing, the difficulties of dealing
> with details of work in the hospital, and the peculiarities
> of certain teachers and departments.

Such remarks apply equally well to the recurrent preoccupations and problems of the Edinburgh students. The choice and 'evaluation' of clinical units is almost exclusively a matter of student culture, and is all but totally based on information shared within the student body. (One or two students from Edinburgh medical families have additional sources of information: they can obtain 'inside knowledge' which otherwise is usually unavailable).

At the outset, of course, the fourth year students all lack firsthand experience of any clinical units. In order to acquire reliable 'tips', they must look to those who have already been through that part of the course, and who therefore 'know the ropes' (cf. Geer et al., 1968).

They look to students in the fifth and sixth years to advise them on the best course of action, and as to the relevant criteria in judging units and evaluating their educational experience. In this way the accumulated 'folk wisdom' of the student culture is passed on from cohort to cohort.

As the year unfolds the fourth years begin to have their own experience to exchange. Indeed, from the very first day on the wards, they enthusiastically swap anecdotes and evaluations about their patients, their teachers and the organisation of their clinical work. As they meet informally after teaching, the students compare notes about their own progress, and about the qualities of their respective cliniques. The students are thus engaged, at an informal level, in a process of 'continuous assessment' of their teachers and teaching.

This is not to imply that there is complete consensus within the student culture. Some cliniques are almost universally approved of: others are pretty well unanimously regarded as poor. But there are many instances where opinions differ as to the relative merits of different clinical units. For the student seeking advice it is often a matter of 'you pays your money and you takes your choice'. The students recognise that the whole process can be something of a lottery. Some indeed opt out of the business of information seeking and sharing: they pick their attachments with a pin, as it were.

Collectively, then, the students are actively engaged in monitoring the educational experience offered in the various cliniques. Individually, they plan their passage through their various attachments, and evaluate them as they progress. They judge what they refer to as the 'atmosphere' of cliniques, a general student term which embraces a number of evaluative criteria.

In organising their evaluations of different clinical units, the students use a sort of 'folk taxonomy' (cf. Atkinson, 1977). The major discrimination which students use to differentiate cliniques is, unsurprisingly, the contrast between Medicine and Surgery. Throughout the year they draw parallels and contrasts between the two specialties. In addition, they divide the teaching hospitals into two types: 'central' and 'peripheral'. In the broader context this latter pair of terms is a relative one: a hospital which is regarded as 'central' from one point of view may be seen as 'peripheral' from another. Thus in comparison with hospitals in outlying areas all the Edinburgh hospitals may be called 'central'. But when they differentiate between the Edinburgh hospitals, students refer to the Royal Infirmary as the 'centre', and to the other teaching hospitals as 'peripheral'. A further distinction is drawn between 'professorial' and 'non-professorial' units. In the former, the clinical staff are University employees, and they are headed by a professor; they hold honorary NHS appointments. The non-professorial units are staffed by NHS clinicians, who may hold honorary University posts.

The students use these dimensions to generate their own 'map' of the relevant portions of the medical school. While the categories of unit are based on aspects of the formal organisation of the school and the hospitals, the students endow them with their own, informal, connotations. It is believed that while each clinique has its own unique 'atmosphere', they vary systematically in accordance with these

dimensions. The students offer each other generalisations: 'all
surgical units are....'; 'peripheral hospitals tend to....'; 'you'll
find that the professorial cliniques are more....'. On the basis of
such typifications students seek out likely cliniques for their own
training. They also attempt to relate the typical expectations of the
student culture to their own past and present experiences of individual
cliniques.

STAFF AND STUDENTS

As in other educational milieux, their relationships with staff members
is an important element in the students' evaluations of clinique
'atmosphere'. For these junior students, their working relations with
clinical staff, especially consultants, are of particular moment, and
are, potentially, fraught.

  In the first place, the clinical teachers are themselves practitioners,
and are potential superiors in students' subsequent work. Even if
individual members of staff are not seen as likely 'hirers and firers',
they nevertheless occupy the position of superiors in the professional
hierarchy. (Some individual consultants, of course, may stand very
high in the medical pantheon). Similarly, the 'reality-like' nature of
clinical instruction means that the teacher student relationships may be
taken by both sides to approximate to a working relationship. All in
all, consultants in medicine and surgery in the teaching hospitals may
present a daunting prospect to young novices.

  The clinical teaching often takes place in a charged atmosphere. That
is, the small group teaching sessions can be quite demanding on the
students. They are 'in play' for the duration of the teaching, and may
be called on to 'perform' before their peers, the clinician and the
patient, in taking a history and performing an examination. The
students may be 'grilled' on their medical knowledge, also in this semi
public fashion. While one should not over dramatise the extent to which
the students are 'on trial', it does give an edge to their day to day
relations with clinicians - particularly the more senior members of
staff.

  For these junior students, the exposure to clinical medicine, real
patients and clinical teachers, is a potentially threatening experience.
The 'atmosphere' which is created and sustained on a clinical unit is
therefore a critical consideration for them. It is possible for a
clinician to make life extremely uncomfortable for students. They have
available to them, for instance, the technique of 'showing them up'
(Woods, 1975) before the patients and their peers. As Wood shows
(admittedly in a very different educational context) students are
vulnerable to the weapons of sarcasm, humiliation and degradation. To
give just one extreme example: I observed one rather irascible
consultant physician respond in this way to a student he regarded as
having performed ineptly:

  'What's your name?'

  'Reid, sir'.

  'And where do <u>reeds</u> grow? In dark wet places - you idiot!'

(I have changed the student's name in such a way as to preserve the force of the consultant's pun). Such extreme tongue lashings are, of course, rare, and seldom so venomous. But students are frequently, and understandably, reluctant to show themselves up, or to be shown up. Bedside interaction, then, can be tense for the potentially incompetent student (cf. Haas and Shaffir, 1977).

Students are also concerned with their incorporation and involvement into the 'team' of clinical staff on the wards. On entering the first clinical year, the students have crossed a major divide in their careers, and have, in some degree, entered the 'real world' of clinical hospital medicine. In the course of their clinical instruction, the students' perspective is that of the doctors, rather than that of other health workers on the ward. Yet the students are not doctors themselves. They do not perform the same tasks, do not have comparable responsibilities, functions or status. Their position is therefore an ambiguous one, poised somewhat uncertainly between the 'lay' world and the medical world of their teachers. Their involvement in the wards is only temporary and part time: they are subordinate and marginal. Yet, for the most part, they would like to be made to feel 'a part of things'. Hence the precise nature of students' relations with their clinical instructors can assume a critical significance in the development of their self perceptions and their evaluation of clinical 'atmosphere'.

The fourth year students therefore pay close attention to their position vis-a-vis the doctors on their attachments. There are two related issues. The first concerns the degree of personal contact between clinicians and students. Despite their close proximity to the clinicians, the actual teaching can come over as anonymous and impersonal. Especially in units where a large number of doctors have teaching responsibilities, students may find that they remain unknown as individuals. The learning of their names by staff, for instance, is one indicator used to gauge the staff's interest in students and the degree of 'colleagueship' that is established. For example, in characterising a surgical unit unfavourably, one student remarked, 'Mr Williams is the only one who's bothered to learn names'; by · contrast, the feeling (rightly or wrongly) was that the other surgeons had not 'bothered' to identify the students as individuals.

As this suggests, the students also attempt to judge the staff members' interest in teaching them. They recognise that clinical teaching is only one of a number of calls on a physician's or a surgeon's time - including routine patient care, research and administration. They appreciate the competing demands on their time and energy. They are mindful too that for junior staff there may be the pressure of their own training and work for 'Fellowship' or 'Membership' examinations. But they get the impression that the degree of commitment displayed towards the teaching of fourth years varies considerably from doctor to doctor, and from unit to unit. For instance:

Jane told me she had applied to wards____ and ____ : but she had been down there with Frances (her flatmate and another fourth year medical student) to see one of the surgeons there. He had said, 'Oh, do we have to do all that teaching again?' She obviously took this to indicate a lack of interest in the teaching programme. She added that she understood surgeons had been telling the students

to go away and read things up in the Medical Reading Room,
rather than teaching them.

Students therefore employ this criterion in categorising clinique
'atmosphere'. For instance, I asked one student what sort of thing he
went on in choosing cliniques:

> Well, the report of the teaching; and sort of how organised
> it is and how interested they seem in teaching the students.
> 'Cos I mean some units, they don't - they'd rather get on
> with ward work rather than teach students, and in others
> they're very pleased to see you. Teaching is something they
> quite enjoy, probably because it provides them with a bit of
> amusement as well when you do something wrong.

This evaluation is often used to discriminate between medicine and
surgery. It is a frequently voiced typification that the surgeons
often appear 'uninterested' or 'uninvolved' in their work with the
junior students. For example, as students told me:

> Both medicine wards have been very good though emotionally
> traumatic. Surgery was poor - the staff seemed very
> uninterested.

> On [surgical unit] I don't think I really got to know the
> staff, or that they took very much interest in us, in
> comparison with the last place [a medical unit].

The nature of staff student relationships is also used to distinguish
between units in the 'centre' and in the 'periphery'. The clinical
teachers at 'the Royal' are thought, on the whole, to expect a greater
degree of formality and to encourage a greater social distance between
themselves and the students. Clinicians in other hospitals (especially
physicians) are thought to foster a much more 'relaxed' atmosphere.

The degree of 'friendliness' and 'colleagueship' which students feel
in their relations with clinicians is also felt to be a reflection of
the quality of working relationships between the ward personnel
themselves. The 'central' units of the Royal Infirmary are believed to
have a particularly 'competitive' ethos. Although the students report
that they enjoy good relationships with junior staff in 'the Royal',
they also feel that these younger physicians and surgeons are acutely
aware of their own career contingencies. The Infirmary is seen as that
part of the medical school which enjoys the highest prestige, thus
recruiting the ablest and most ambitious young men and women (though
there are few enough of the latter). The students therefore feel that
these junior doctors are involved in a 'rat race' (as many of them
phrased it), competing for recognition, jealous of each other's research
productivity, and jostling for the consultant's attention. Whether or
not the students are correct in thinking that this is particularly acute
in the Infirmary, it is certainly the case that generally there is a
great deal of competition for promotion in such popular hospital
specialties as medicine and surgery.

Competition is also felt to characterise the professional
relationships of the more senior staff members. It is argued that in
the 'peripheral' hospitals, the consultant staff enjoy friendly

relations, whereas this intimacy is lacking in the more 'formal' atmosphere of the Royal Infirmary. At the same time the consultants at 'the Royal' are thought to compete with each other, in terms of their professional standing, their expertise, and the treatment of esoteric conditions. (I have no direct information on the actual quality of professional relations. But it must be pointed out that the Infirmary is a good deal larger and more complex organisation than the so called 'peripheral' hospitals, where greater intimacy may be more readily achieved).

Although relationships among the staff do not normally impinge directly on the fourth year students, the students themselves take this aspect of ward life as a reflection of the more general and pervasive ethos of a given clinical unit. Indeed, this atmosphere is felt to colour the attitudes of nursing staff. Admittedly, the junior students do not have all that much direct contact with the nurses. But they do form impressions of the nurses' attitudes towards students. For instance, they judge whether the nurses regard students as an unwelcome intrusion on the wards (or at least whether they express such reservations by word or deed).

In all these ways, then, the fourth year students attempt to make sense of their introduction on to the hospital wards, and to judge the extent to which they are granted some degree of 'colleagueship' by their clinical teachers. These concerns are parallelled by comparable interests in their relations with the hospital patients.

RELATIONS WITH PATIENTS

For the fourth year students it is the outstanding feature of their introduction to clinical work that they begin to work with actual patients. Such patient contact is the touchstone of the authenticity of their medical experience. It is also crucial to their own developing self perception as young doctors in the making. At the same time they are concerned to monitor not only their own interaction with patients, but also those of their teachers (cf. Dowling and Cotsonas, 1964). They expect the clinicians, ideally, to treat their patients in a 'considerate' and 'humanitarian' fashion.

There has been a long standing interest in the 'idealism' or 'cynicism' of medical students and other professionals in training. One version of the argument suggests that students begin with a predisposition towards idealism: in the course of their professional training, that character trait is gradually replaced by one of cynicism (e.g. Eron, 1955). An alternative view suggests that this apparent change is not a matter of psychological characteristics. Rather, it is seen as a reflection of situational factors. That is, a display of 'cynicism', or something like it, is a part of medical school culture: it is the 'done thing' to express such attitudes, at least in public, this latter view proposes, but that does not necessarily reveal fundamental changes in attitude (e.g. Becker and Geer, 1958).

That argument is primarily one about socialisation, about the effect of medical school over time. It is, of course, more than that: it reflects competing theories and methodologies, as well as honest to goodness conceptual muddle). In the nature of things the research reported here cannot deal with such change directly. It was, however, noticeable that the students did employ notions which might be called 'idealistic' (though one of the conceptual problems I referred to is the fact that 'idealism' and 'cynicism' gloss over a legion of possible attitudes, vocabularies of motive and so on). The fourth year students recognise that in order to survive as a medical student, one had to 'harden' oneself; that it would be no use to be squeamish or emotionally vulnerable. Nevertheless they expect to be able to establish sympathetic relationships with their patients, and to preserve a degree of what Lief and Fox (1963) call 'detached concern'. They expect their clinical teachers to display the same concern, and they judge them accordingly. They do not find that the doctors are all equally 'humane' in their approach (or at least, do not appear to be so).

Among other things, the students use this criterion to distinguish between the typical features of their experiences in medicine and surgery. It is a commonly voiced criticism of surgery that the observed relationships between the surgeons and their patients are not as satisfying as those pertaining between the physicians and their patients. The surgeons appear to place much less emphasis on the interpersonal aspects of their patient care.

According to this view, the surgeons come over to their students as more 'callous', 'brusque' or 'offhand' with their patients. They seem to approach their work with a much more limited focus than do the physicians. They are often seen as concentrating more on the purely physical aspects of patient care - with the technicalities of surgery itself - than on the care and well-being of the 'whole patient'. Students hold up the ideal of treating each patient individually, as a 'person' rather than as a 'case', and the majority find the surgeons lacking. (As is usually the case with such stereotyping, the student view does not explicate what would actually be implied by 'treating patients as people'). Some students argue vigorously on the surgeon's behalf, maintaining that the stereotype is false - that surgeons are not really callous, and practise a type of medicine every bit as good as that practised by the physicians. Yet even these defenders acknowledge the potency of the negative stereotype among their classmates. Certainly the detractors of surgery are in the majority. Rightly or wrongly they voice the criticism that the surgeons tend to see patients primarily as 'a lump' or 'a stomach' rather than as 'Mr or Mrs So and so'. As an indicator of this attitude, the students claim to observe that surgeons remember their patients' names less often than the physicians.

This criterion is also drawn on in the students' comparison of 'central' and 'peripheral' units. The more 'impersonal' atmosphere which they associate with 'the Royal' is felt to colour doctor patient relationships. The students' folk wisdom has it that, for both medicine and surgery, the peripheral units tend towards a more 'patient centred' approach to practice. The 'central' firms, on the other hand, are held to exemplify a contrasting medical ideology. The doctors on such units are generally believed to concentrate their efforts on more 'technological' or 'scientific' styles, at the expense of patient oriented medicine. They are said to be more interested in academic, research oriented work.

The students' expectations and perceptions of their own patient
contacts mirror their ideas about doctor patient relationships. There
is a sharp difference between medicine and surgery in this respect. In
keeping with the views outlined above, the students' experience is that
they themselves are able to form more and closer relations with patients
on the medical ward than they are on surgery. As I have already
indicated, the opportunity to work with patients on the ward is an
especially salient feature of the students' experience, and the
opportunity to engage in such clinical work is highly valued.
Consequently the fourth year students judge the various clinical firms
in terms of the scope they offer for working directly with patients, and
thus of accumulating personal experience of something they regard as
central to 'real' clinical medicine.

Most medical units are felt to offer adequate opportunity for such
experience to be acquired. A relatively high proportion of the time is
spent in bedside teaching, and there is correspondingly less emphasis
on tutorials or lectures in the unit's teaching room. While attached to
medical wards, therefore, students are able to feel that they spend more
of their time at the 'coal face' of clinical practice. At this early
stage in the clinical phase of their undergraduate training, it is
understandable that work with patients should have such a high value, if
only in terms of novelty - in addition to its value in symbolising
'authentic' medicine. The opportunity to 'clerk' patients is probably
the most highly prized clinical opportunity of this sort. Students can
then work with an individual patient over a more protracted period than
is usually possible - often spread over several days. Working alone,
taking a full history and completing a thorough physical examination,
the students feel that they are able to achieve the degree of
acquaintance and rapport which they value. Moreover, this exercise
approximates most closely the actual clinical work performed by the
doctors. Students are normally expected to write up 'their' case(s),
outlining the main findings, and essaying differential diagnosis. Such
a product - the case notes - is tangible evidence of the 'real' clinical
work the students put in, and its production mimics the actual work put
in by the medical staff on admitting a patient.

The students' initial experience of such clinical matters (gained on
medical units in the first term of the year) is treasured as a major
step forward in their accumulation of relevant experience. When they
progress to a surgical attachment in the second or third term, they
often find themselves disappointed. There is, they report, less scope
for such contact with patients. There is, in the first place, more
emphasis on lectures or seminars, less on bedside teaching and ward
rounds. Secondly, there is less opportunity to 'clerk' patients and
follow through individual cases. Consequently, the students tend to
evaluate surgical units negatively and to compare them unfavourably
with their medical attachments. They grumble that they lack sufficient
contact with the patients, have little chance to take a detailed case
history or perform a systematic physical examination. They complain too
that while they are on the surgical wards they have insufficient time to
practise their new clinical skills. The techniques which they have so
dearly acquired during their introductory week are, they maintain,
'getting rusty'. Furthermore, this lack of patient contact robs the
students of opportunities to experience their emerging identities as
'doctors' in the context of 'real' patient care.

DETECTIVE WORK

There is one aspect of clinical work which the students appreciate in particular. They often refer to it as 'detective work'. The task of history taking, examination and differential diagnosis presents the students with something which is, potentially, a satisfying and stimulating intellectual exercise. Thus students learn to spot the distinctive, pathognomic indications of particular diseases, and the skills necessary to elicit relevant clinical information. Their clinical teachers encourage the use of the 'special senses', exhorting the students to use their powers of observation and inference to the full. Occasionally, they are encouraged to make an 'end-of-the bed' spot diagnosis on the basis of some readily observable clinical sign. On other occasions, the students need to piece together more complex information, perhaps called from different sources (the clinical findings, test results, X-ray plates etc.). However it is done, this process of diagnosis is highly valued and success at it a source of some pride. As I have indicated the students liken it to the work of the detective. (It is worth remembering that in creating the character of Sherlock Holmes Conan Doyle took as his model an Edinburgh doctor, and based his famous technique of detection on the doctor's teaching methods).

This sort of inquiry and reasoning is associated particularly with internal medicine, which is therefore seen as a more enjoyable and absorbing enterprise: the concerns of surgery, on the other hand, are seen to be much more limited - the surgeons' work being more restricted in intellectual and practical scope. Many of the students formulate a stereotype in which the surgeon's diagnostic task is less demanding than the physician's. He may have to be no more precise than to identify an 'acute abdomen', and then he can 'go in' and 'have a look'. He can deal directly with the patient's condition, whereas the physician has to work 'at a distance'. Whereas the physician has to rely on his clinical inference, the surgeon can, in the last resort, confirm his hunches by direct observation. As one student put it:

> Surgery is very limited intellectually. You can make a
> diagnosis, but it's not so crucially important because
> in the end you're going to cut the patient up anyway,
> and find out whether you're right or wrong.

At their least charitable the students claim that the surgeon is more of a technician or craftsman ('a carpenter' is a frequent epithet). He is seen as a manual worker, as opposed to the more cerebral physician. Similarly, surgeons are said to work mainly on rather specific, localised disease (a fact which contributes to their treatment of patients as 'cases'). The problems of internal medicine are often more general and more diffuse, making greater demands on the physicians' clinical acumen.

It probably goes without saying that this view of surgery is not one with which most surgeons would agree, and it is not the image which they consciously project for the specialty in their teaching. There is a small minority of students who do not subscribe to the popular stereotype: they find in surgery intellectual challenge and satisfaction, and defend the specialty against the detractors. In particular they take issue with the belief that surgery is limited intellectually, and point out the complexities of post operative care, as well as the sheer technical expertise involved in its practice.

It might well be thought that surgery would offer its own compensating advantages to the fourth year students. Generally speaking, surgery has a glamour all of its own - not least in the drama and tension of the operating theatre. Such, at least, is the popular view of this branch of medicine. One might reasonably expect the fourth year students to be pleased and even enthusiastic at the idea of direct exposure to surgical operations.

To some extent this is the case. Certainly at the very outset the students do appreciate the chance to observe the surgeons at work in the theatre. As with other aspects of clinical work, students gain the impression that they are participating in the 'reality' of hospital medicine. The first operations which students observe are treated as landmarks in their growing clinical experience. But for many of them the novelty soon wears off. The reason for this is not hard to find. As very junior novices, the students' role in surgery must always be that of a passive observer of the scene rather than that of active participant. For the most part, there is little for a group of up to twelve students to do other than watch an operation from an observation gallery. Ultimately then, the students' distance from and non involvement in the surgical work is emphasised. Their junior status is reinforced, and they rarely feel incorporated as 'junior colleagues'.

'Waiting nights', on the other hand, do provide some opportunity for students to gain experience of more direct involvement. Since they normally attend in small numbers (usually a couple at a time) it is much more feasible for the fourth year students to become much more involved with the work of the surgeons. They can see patients admitted, and are often able to follow them through into theatre. At such times the one or two fourth years present have a much better chance of observing the surgery at close quarters. If they are lucky they also get the chance to 'assist' at operations (in practice, holding a retractor). This sort of participation is viewed very positively. But such occasions tend to be rare 'treats', in comparison with routine instruction in surgery.

Students do prize operations which they have observed at close hand or at which they have assisted. Be it only a minor operation - for haemarrhoids, or a circumcision, say - the first few are highly significant 'benchmarks' in the collection of clinical experience. They are recounted by students to their friends, with not a little personal pride. (Obviously this only 'works' during these early days of clinical training. Later in their careers they would hardly be able to boast of having been present at a circumcision).

One of the 'central' surgical units I observed has an arrangement whereby a small group of students in the clinique can attend a small 'peripheral' hospital for part of their attachment. There it is possible for them to be more directly involved in the day to day work of the surgeons there. There is a remarkable contrast between the students' enthusiasm for this brief period of their work and their relative indifference towards their work on the 'proper' unit. They are eager to recount their experiences in the 'periphery', and to catalogue the operations (not in themselves very serious or 'dramatic') which they had closely observed or assisted at. Their experience serves to highlight that of the majority of students who do not have an equivalent opportunity.

WORK AND EFFORT

The likely 'level' of effort expected in different firms is another of the concerns shared by the fourth year students. So too is the 'direction' of their effort. (On 'level and direction of effort', cf. Becker et al., 1961). In other words they are preoccupied with the amount of work and effort demanded from them, and the sort of tasks at which they are required to work. (This sort of concern was also one of the most, if not the single most, pressing of the topics dealt with by the student culture at the Kansas medical school). As one might expect, the various cliniques, by virtue of their different approaches to medicine or surgery, and their different commitments to teaching, are seen to demand varying degrees of effort on the students' part.

It is by no means the case, however, that students seek out, or appreciate, those clinical firms which are thought to have low expectations of their students or low levels of 'productivity'. On the contrary, those units which are identified as 'lazy' in their approach are avoided if possible for that very reason. Some students in fact appear to be almost masochistic in this respect - expecting to be worked hard on their clinical attachments and annoyed if they are not. As I have indicated already, the first year of clinical study is seen as less gruelling than the traumatic preparation for the '2nd MB' at the end of the previous year. And the students are grateful for that, but they certainly do not value too easy a ride.

This perspective derives from a rational calculation (and of course has nothing to do with masochism really). They recognise that the experience gained in the fourth year will be a most important grounding in the basics of clinical work. They are therefore justifiably concerned that, given the apparent variability of cliniques, they should find themselves attached to ones which prepare them adequately and expose them to the necessary range of experience in sufficient depth. This has a bearing on their training and on their careers in general. The fourth year is the time when they should be laying the foundations of sound technique, basic knowledge and so on. They are also concerned with shorter term issues. They need to make sure that they are adequately prepared and 'covered' for the clinical examinations at the end of the year. One 'atrocity story' (Stimson and Webb, 197) which was circulated at the time of the fieldwork was related about a certain surgical unit. It was claimed that all those who had been there had failed surgery in the summer examinations. The unit was avoided on those grounds, and it was held up as a dreadful warning against a careless choice of clinique. (During the fieldwork itself there was no evidence of such a correlation between specific attachments and examination failures: but these myths defy such sober facts).

In fact it is not at all easy for students to evaluate whether they have achieved the appropriate experience and mastery. There is no precisely defined syllabus for the clinical instruction. There are broad aims which are clearly recognised: the development of competence in the basic skills such as history taking and examination, and an ability to recognise the signs and symptoms of a variety of diseases. But there is no specific indication of what fourth year students should have done, should have witnessed, or should know about. Consequently, their evaluation of their progress must take place in something of a vacuum. A constant comparison of one's own range of experience against that of other students is therefore of considerable importance.

The fact that the 'curriculum' of clinical instruction remains to a considerable extent unwritten and implicity is in large measure a direct reflection of the basic character of such clinical work. It must depend very largely on the routine practice of the units concerned, the availability of patients with relevant disorders and so on. In the nature of things, the exact nature and timing of clinical work is unpredictable and it would not normally be possible for it to be specified in detail in advance. Clinicians cannot readily legislate for the presence and sequence of patients who may come under their care. The actual content of a student's experience on any individual clinique, and hence over the entire year, is uncertain. All the information which students have to go in planning an undergraduate career, and in evaluating their progress rests on the shared stock of knowledge and experience enshrined in the student culture.

The foregoing considerations do not mean that all students go flat out to attend units which demand the very highest effort. For the most part they week to balance the level of effort. Some individual clinicians, or their firms, are felt to be too demanding.

As I have emphasised, the first days on the wards constitute a major transition in the students' careers: while welcomed, it is an experience which brings its own demands. The novelty of the setting, the acquisition of new skills, the exposure to patients, are all felt to be potentially stressful. The first contacts with patients can seem, by turns, exciting, traumatic, enjoyable or depressing. Hence many of the students appreciate what they describe as a 'fairly gentle' introduction to this uncharted territory, in an atmosphere which is not too taxing on their intellectual and emotional resources. Cliniques are valued insofar as they provide a 'relaxed' atmosphere for the introduction to clinical studies.

Cliniques which are not 'relaxed' are described as 'high powered'. In terms of students' typifications, the 'central' cliniques in the Royal Infirmary are felt to be more 'high powered' than those in the 'periphery' (a view which is in keeping with the other perceptions of clinique atmosphere already outlined). The staff at the Royal are believed to expect more of their students, in terms of the amount of new material they are required to assimilate, the pace of the teaching, and the amount of formal instruction provided. (In fact there is rather more time available for teaching at the Royal Infirmary than elsewhere: some time is lost in 'bussing' the students to 'peripheral' hospitals). The typical sort of comment offered about the experience of the Royal is that students there are 'thrown in at the deep end' of clinical work. Units elsewhere are described as providing a more gradual start. For example:

Over coffee it came out that the students had gathered there are differences between the [peripheral] Hospital and the

Royal Infirmary. They told me that they were being introduced
to clinical experience 'fairly gently', whilst those at the
Infirmary were being 'pushed in at the deep end'.

Over and above the fact that the majority of them are 'central', the
professorial units are said to be particularly 'high powered'. This is
in accordance with their perceived 'academic' orientation. Professorial
units are thought of as being especially demanding, and to exercise
exceptionally strong control over the students' work. Their
distinctive atmosphere is sometimes spoken of as 'hot house'. For this
reason, some students try to avoid units of this sort. The hot house
atmosphere is related to the competitiveness which students believe
characterises such academic settings: in the face of such (supposed)
competition and rivalry, the staff members' demeanour is held to imply a
display of superior academic fire power, as the clinicians vie for
kudos.

The students are also keen to gain general experience, rather than
being exposed to an overspecialised and restricted range of clinical
matters. In broad terms all the firms which students attend are
general, but 'some are more general than others'. Students sometimes
grumble that their introduction to clinical medicine or surgery is
imbalanced because their clinical teachers spend too much time on their
specialised work. On one surgical unit, for instance, students grumbled
that they knew 'all there is to know about colostomies', but had not
covered other aspects of more general interest. In this context, too,
then the students are interested in a close evaluation of the quality of
educational experience which they acquire in the course of their
attachment to various clinical firms in the teaching hospitals.

CLINIQUES AND CAREERS

In addition to the need for the immediate choice of fourth year units,
there may be significant considerations to be born in mind concerning
future contingencies. This arises from the element of 'patronage' in
the organisation of medical careers (cf. Hall, 1948), which is of
crucial relevance at the end of the students' undergraduate course,
when they must seek posts as house-physicians and house-surgeons during
their 'pre-registration' year.

The particular hospitals and clinical firms where a student undertakes
this year of work can be of considerable importance in the development
of his or her subsequent career and attainment within medicine. To
complete a house job successfully in a teaching hospital which enjoys
high prestige is an important first step on the ladder of a successful
career in the medical profession. Similarly, to be employed in the
'firm' of a well known and important consultant is an important career
contingency.

For a student with any degree of ambition, then, the prospect of
obtaining a favourable house job in one of the popular firms in an
Edinburgh teaching hospital is a consideration to be borne in mind. It
may be seen as an important goal to be attained at the end of the
student's undergraduate career. Not all the fourth year students
actively consider their pre-registration year, but of those who do the
majority believe that it is desirable to complete at least one of the

house jobs in one of Edinburgh's hospitals. To leave and go elsewhere might look less well in the future: it might suggest that one has not been considered good enough to be offered a post by any of the clinicians who have a close personal knowledge of one's work as a student. One of the male students I talked to articulated this concern, and I summarised our conversation in my field notes:

> For his pre-registration year he would probably stay in Edinburgh, and at the moment the [peripheral] hospital was an appealing proposition. Staying in Edinburgh was important, otherwise, when one is applying for jobs, people would ask you why you didn't do a house job in your teaching area. On the whole he thought this was unfortunate, as he would like to move about more freely ....He said that when consultants are looking for housemen to look after their patients they will naturally prefer the student they know; they will therefore be most likely to take someone who has worked under them for a final year attachment. He added, 'Maybe it's just an old boy tradition'. He repeated that one's final year attachments are important for where you do your house job....Some people, he told me, even get their house jobs fixed very early, even immediately after their summer clerkships. He also told me that there is more care taken over Final Phase attachments than in choosing junior cliniques.

The selection of successful candidates for house jobs, as the students see it, depends very largely on their personal relationships with the consultant staff of their Final Phase units. The jobs are seen as being largely in the hands of the chief of the firm, and the successful application for a job could depend on a student's being 'well in' with the clinicians concerned.

Future success in medicine is therefore seen to depend largely on creating a good impression with a consultant under whom one would like to train during one's first postgraduate year, and perhaps subsequently, should one become a senior house officer, registrar and so on. In other words, the most advantageous transition to postgraduate teaching is seen by the students as being a process of 'sponsored mobility' (Turner, 1960). In order to maximise one's chances of such sponsorship and recruitment, it may be necessary to manage one's 'self presentation' with some care (cf. Goffman, 1971). 'Impression management' on the part of the students can therefore be geared towards creating a favourable impression with staff members, as prospective sponsors and professional superiors. For instance, after a conversation with two students,(one male, one female), I noted:

> They both agreed that getting on in a speciality depended on what one of them called 'the coefficient between ability and getting on with the clinical staff'. You can, one of them said, be a surgeon of moderate ability and yet be successful because 'you happen to click with a surgeon', or you can be a very good surgeon and fail to get on because of poor relations with members of staff.

These students were expecting this 'coefficient' to be of importance in their later experiences in the medical school, and in their subsequent careers, should they find themselves committed to a career in a hospital speciality. Another male student I interviewed was similarly explicit about the process, although he wished to disassociate himself from the practice of impression management:

St. People feel it's time to impress people. There's a lot of this goes on, I don't really like it.

P.A. What do people do?

St. The occasional 'sir', being nice, not being obstreperous, being benign and harmless.

He added that he suspected that a lot of clinicians could 'see through' this sort of impression management on the students' part, so that it was not always totally effective. He also stressed that it was not really an effective strategy at the fourth year stage, being more relevant for the students in their final year.

St. You try to pick a final year attachment where you want to do a house job, and then you turn on the charm.

Just as this student sought to distance himself from these practices, so do many of his peers. An awareness of this career strategy is admitted to by many students, but it is something that is generally attributed to others; it is 'something that goes on' rather than 'something we do'. Students are reticent about appearing over keen or 'pushy' in the eyes of the fellow members of the clinique. During the fourth year, competition for attention and recognition is not pressing. To push oneself forward at this stage may be to risk contravention of the students' collective levels and directions of effort. But as the following extract from my field notes suggests, this consideration may be oriented to by students in their interaction with clinicians:

The group were discussion whether or not they were going to go and hear their chief, who was giving that week's clinical lecture for the final hour that morning. Roy Bateson was in a bad mood and seemed genuinely unwilling to go along. One of his fellow students said he reckoned that it all depended on whether he wanted to 'keep in' with Dr Crosbie, with an eye to his future career.

The implication of this was that the student's absence from the lecture might well be noted by the chief, and might be remembered and held against him subsequently. This group of students were in fact approaching the matter in a fairly light hearted way. Nevertheless, they did appear to be voicing a genuine concern over career management.

One student in particular drew attention to the importance of the 'informal' criteria which students may have to bear in mind in thinking about their careers, and their implications for practice beyond qualification. Our conversation had turned to why people opt for an 'honours year':

St. I think the major reason people go into them is that they realise that it'll help them get a job later.

P.A.   Is that true?

St.   Well I think, I mean, we're all churned out at the same
       level: you know there's no classes in the MB ChB, so I
       think if you've got other things that you can add on,
       like honours Pathology or something, it'll help you get
       a good post. There's a lot of other ways of doing it
       though. One of the most recent ones I've heard of in
       the final year if you do a locum, a week or so, it gets
       you well known and well liked. That's when you do it
       well, of course; if you kill a patient they're not
       going to be too happy.

As this student so well describes, there is a recurrent problem
facing the career conscious student. As one of a large number of
students he finds himself relatively anonymous. Few can reasonably
expect to be outstanding academically and to impress members of staff on
their examination performances alone. Yet the allocation of first
hospital posts is often felt to depend upon the personal choice of the
consultants on the various wards. As one student told me, 'It depends
largely on how many people you impress' as to how successful a student
is in his or her applications for house posts. As is apparent in the
extracts I have already quoted, students do not deny the relevance of
academic ability and qualifications (honours degrees and distinctions in
examinations are recognised as depending upon intellectual ability).
Rather, they suggest that in themselves they may not be sufficient
conditions for success, however necessary. Ability must be matched by
careful career management and some success in 'fronting' (cf. Olesen and
Whittaker, 1968, p.173 ff.). For students of average or below average
academic attainment in the medical school, then 'fronting' will be a
major recourse.

Whilst these considerations 'filter down' to students in the fourth
year, the topic of house jobs impinges on their immediate plans in a
rather indirect way. To be precise, it informs a strategy of avoiding
certain units rather than seeking them out. The rationality for this
procedure is derived from a simple rule. That is, that in the normal
run of events, students are not admitted to units for their final year
attachments if they have already been there for their fourth year
teaching. In other words, attachment to a clinical unit for a fourth
year clinique will normally preclude attachment to that same unit in
the student's last year. The students' strategies of clinique choice
are (or may be) formulated with this in mind.

There may, therefore, be some conflict in students' decision making.
They need to reconcile the dilemma of opting directly for popular and
attractive units, and deliberately avoiding them in the hope of being
able to obtain an attachment in one or more of them in their final year
(when the 'pay off' may be of greater and more lasting significance).
In other words, a strongly fancied unit may not be put down as a
preference, but may be 'saved up' for the later part of the
undergraduate course. During the closing weeks of my second term's
observation, for instance, I noted students employing this tactic in
coming to decisions about clinique choices for the coming term:

    I overheard a fifth year girl giving another girl advice about
    possible attachments to try for in her term of surgery. She

named two of these possible cliniques, but added that her
friend should do her best to keep one of them back for
her final year attachment.

Similarly, in discussing how she had chosen her first medical unit,
one of the female students told me that in doing so, she had 'done a bit
of asking around' with students in the year above her. They had told
her that the unit she picked would offer her 'a good start' in clinical
medicine.

This aspect of clinique choice was also displayed by other students
during the year:

Gerald Kennedy had deliberately steered clear of
[peripheral] Hospital, so that for his final year his
chances are good for getting an attachment there. He
explained that you have to do eight weeks in the Royal
Infirmary anyway, so it is a good idea to keep options
open for the peripheral units. His general planning
is to be in the [peripheral] Hospital, as he would like
to get a house job there....The___Hospital is 'no good
to anybody', and as for the ____Hospital, 'you have to
be a certain type, beer swilling and back slapping'.

One of the female students I interviewed also articulated this concern:

P.A.   How did you pick [her present unit]?

St.   It was mainly...going on previous reports. The
       fact that I didn't want to come to the Royal
       until the last term, but I didn't want to come
       to the [peripheral] again, 'cos I wanted to
       leave various options open for the final year.
       It's all a question of fiddling things, isn't it?

If students should fail to obtain an attachment to the units of their
preference in the first clinical year, or if they discover that a
chosen unit does not suit them, or is not all its reputation led them
to expect, then the perspective of 'deferred gratification' can be
turned to good account. While present experience may be judged
unsatisfactory, students can reconcile themselves to this by the thought
that at least it is now 'out of the way'. The rule against returning to
a fourth year unit can therefore be seen to protect the student against
having to repeat the experience. This can be illustrated from my field
notes. During a coffee time conversation between two final year
students and a few fourth years, I heard them talking about this aspect
of student careers. They had just been taught by the chief of their
firm, who had been particularly severe and critical with one of the
older students:

A senior, who had been rather picked on by Dr Burton, said
he thought he had been like that because he hadn't wanted
Dr Burton's house job. The conversation turned to house
jobs in general. One of the seniors told the fourth years
that one wants to end up in the Royal for one's final year
attachment (as they had done). The two seniors were in
agreement that the fourth year students were lucky in

having got Dr Burton's attachment 'out of the way' early in
the course. John Cartwright (one of the fourth years) told
them that Dr Burton's firm had been his third choice for
medicine, and he had wanted to do surgery this term anyway.

In such a fashion, apparently 'unlucky' students in the fourth year can
'cool out' their own apparent lack of success. The otherwise poor start
of finding oneself on an unpopular clinique can be reinterpreted as a
fortunate contingency, as an instance of 'luck' rather than the reverse.
In this way the appearance of a favourable and rational career pattern
can be salvaged and reassembled by the employment of the 'deferred
gratification' perspective on cliniques and clinique choices.

COUNTING EXPERIENCE

I have described how students attempt to plan their undergraduate
careers, in order to optimise the experience they gain of clinical work.
I have also described how they evaluate the experience they and their
fellow students actually gain. Since there is no set guide to precisely
what they should encounter, then the students have to engage in a form
of 'research' in order to guage the range of variation. Only in this
way can they place their own individual experience in context. The
'research' strategy they use, and it is one which is familiar to
sociologists, is that of the 'constant comparative method'. On the
basis of their 'folk model' of the teaching hospitals, the students
compare surgical and medical, 'central' and 'peripheral', 'professorial'
and 'non professorial'.

I have outlined some of these student comparisons above, and I have
detailed some of them elsewhere (Atkinson, 1973 and 1974). Here I am
less concerned with the actual detailed comparisons between hospitals
and specialties than with the more general implications of this
'continuous assessment' which fourth year students, individually and
collectively, produce. What they are doing is 'counting clinical
experience'. David Sudnow (1967), in his study of death in hospitals,
provides us with a parallel, and indeed touches on medical education
directly.   In a discussion of how deaths on the ward are treated as
newsworthy, reportable events, Sudnow remarks:

New student nurses and, apparently, young medical students
make it a habit of counting such events as deaths, and
locate their own growing experience and sophistication by
reference to 'how many times' such and such has been
encountered, witnessed, done, etc. Throughout the medical
world, numerical representations of phenomena are accorded
central status as marks of experience. (p.37)

Sudnow goes on to note that there comes a point in one's sophistication
when individual events are no longer counted, when one begins to 'lose
count'.

The fourth year medical students, being novices still, are mostly at
the stage of 'counting' their clinical experiences. Specific events,
and more general features (such as clinique 'atmosphere') are all added
to the store of experience. There is, as I have said, no pre given
corpus of knowledge and experience which the students have to 'put

40

under their belt'. Insofar as they recognise and assemble such a corpus, they have to 'make it up as they go along'. They do, however, come to know that there are many things that they might reasonably learn to do, see done, or at least learn about.

It is a source of great satisfaction to students when they acquire a new experience. (The train spotter offers one analogy here. Another is the stereotypical tourist, who 'does' the approved sights (MacCannell, 1977)). There was, for instance, one student who was in residence at one of the hospitals as a living in 'clerk' (an opportunity available to a few junior students). His duties as a clerk included the collection of blood samples early each morning. He lost no opportunity to drop into conversation references to 'when I was taking bloods this morning ....', and to draw attention to the fact that his fellow students did not share the opportunity for such 'real' clinical experience. On one occasion I came across a student who was quite made up as a result of mistaken identity. A junior doctor had mistaken him for a more senior student, and had asked him to carry out a simple test on one of the patients. He was asked to examine a patient's stool for traces of 'faecal occult blood' (FOB). He had not 'let on' that he was only a fourth year student, and he was clearly very pleased at this opportunity. Ward tasks of this sort are, of course, menial. They are not the sort of thing which the students will continue to carry out eagerly. Indeed they will probably be all too pleased to delegate them to future cohorts of junior students themselves. The students at Kansas (Becker et al., 1961, p.259) complained at being given such 'scut work' to carry out. The novice students at Edinburgh only 'count' such experiences at the outset of their clinical work. But to begin with, they are treasured.

There are many clinical procedures which the students are eager to witness. These include: lumbar punctures; putting up a drip; taking samples of bone marrow; taking blood pressure; passing catheters. If possible they are usually keen to be shown how to do such things, and to practise at least some of them themselves. Such achievements are all 'counted' and recounted to others. In themselves, many of these valued experiences are 'routine', and are the sort of thing which these selfsame students will soon 'lose count of'. By the time they qualify such experiences will have become mundane for them, as they are for all competent and experienced practitioners. For the time being, however, they are far from routine: they are precious novelties. Sometimes students are frustrated, as their teachers may insist on treating these practical accomplishments and spectacles as ordinary, even trivial, and fail to appreciate their significance for the fourth years. The latter, on the other hand, are greedy for experience, and are sometimes afraid that they may find themselves at some future time with major gaps in their basic clinical grounding.

On occasion, some enterprising students use their own initiative to search out extra experience. For instance, one or two make it their business to get to know casualty officers and to visit the Accident and Emergency department in their own time. Here they see 'front line' medicine, much as they do on waiting nights, of a sort very different from what they see during normal bedside teaching. There the students may get the chance to clean, dress and stitch wounds. They are allowed to learn and practise on simple enough injuries, and the casualty officers are no doubt glad enough of their voluntary help.

As I have described already, in addition to these specific clinical experiences, the students evaluate their cliniques in terms of general 'atmosphere'. Crucial to such evaluations is the degree to which the students are made to feel incorporated into the clinical firm, and establish satisfying working relationships with doctors and patients. There has been a debate in the literature on the status of the medical student - whether he or she is to be portrayed as a 'junior colleague', or a 'boy (or girl) in white'. What the Edinburgh students experience is that they enjoy no single status. Sometimes they are treated as junior partners, at other times their passive, marginal position is stressed. (Shuval (1975), makes this point in relation to her research in Israel).

What is important to the fourth year students is the extent to which they can feel part of what is going on on the wards, and can feel that they are, medically speaking, 'where the action is'. Their participation in the 'reality' of the hospital wards and clinics is the touchstone by which their educational and clinical experience is judged. The clinical phase of study is eagerly welcomed on this basis. Although students' ideals are not lived up to equally on all units, their first year of clinical work is, as we have seen, a major turning point. The appeal of the clinical lies in its apparent authenticity, and its rationale in the students' exposure to medical 'reality'.

4 The Clinical Setting

Clinical teaching on the hospital wards, insofar as it derives from an
'apprenticeship' mode of professional socialisation, has features of 'on
the job' training. Although medical students are not working employees
in the organisation, they are taught in the work milieu, in the 'real
world' of medicine. To some extent, as they process round the wards
with a teacher, or work individually whilst 'clerking' patients, the
students are involved in the day to day world of medical work. Yet at
the same time they are not unequivocally members of the ward personnel
and participants in their routine work. It is not so much that they are
incompetent recruits, but rather that the students do not have
responsibility for any aspect of the patient's daily care. Their
position in the hospital is therefore ambiguous. The teaching encounter
at a patient's bedside is to some degree defined as a medical one; in
some ways the work of the teacher and his students is kept distinct from
the rest of the ward and its routine; to some extent therapeutic and
educational work are in competition with each other. This chapter will
explore these facets of the clinical teaching encounter.

The medical milieu and ambiance must be accomplished and sustained as
a prerequisite to the specifically educational tasks at the bedside.
The production of a 'medical' encounter will therefore be considered
first. As Emerson (1970) has pointed out, 'situations differ in how
much effort it takes to sustain the current definition of the
situation', and she cites the gynaecological examination as one which is
extremely precarious. I believe that Emerson attributes specifically to
gynaecological examinations many features that are common to most, if
not all, medical encounters. Certain aspects of medical work require a
degree of careful reality management on the part of medical personnel -
and this applies whether the situation is a 'delicate' internal
examination or a 'straightforward' out patient visit, or indeed a
session with medical students. Emerson comments on a number of reality
sustaining (or creating) devices in her discussion of gynaecologists and
their patients. She points to the fact that the 'medical definition' is
expressed by a number of indicators: that the interaction is located in
a medical milieu, the hospital clinic or doctor's office, for instance.
Within that space decor and equipment complete the medical *mise en
scène*: 'The staff wear medical uniforms, don medical gloves, use medical
instruments'. Similarly, the presence of medical personnel and the
exclusion of lay members 'helps to preclude confusion between the
contact of medicine and the contact of intimacy'.

Emerson also discusses the use of linguistic conventions in
sustaining a medical definition of the situation - for instance, the
substitution of the definite article for pronominal adjective ('the
vagina', not 'your vagina'), or 'delicate' periphasis ('down below' to
refer to the pelvic region, etc.). Along with a degree of impersonality,
Emerson also points out, the examining doctor must attempt to combine
a demeanour suggesting care and concern. She goes on to describe a

number of ways in which such a smooth accomplishment of the examination may be threatened, and further, how such threats may be neutralised by the physician and his nurse, or other attending auxiliary personnel.

I have dwelt at some length on Emerson's description of the gynaecological examination and its routine accomplishment in order to make the following point: *mutatis mutandis* Emerson's description applies equally to most, if not all, medical encounters - and certainly those that take place in a medical locale. In all such encounters the medical ambiance hedges round the actors' construction of reality; in all cases the medical personnel are there, often with paramedical professionals and other auxiliary workers at hand; in all cases the talk and demeanour of the professionals sustains the medical reality. What I am arguing is that Emerson's paper in fact presents a generalised picture of medical reality in a professionalised setting, and I take it as a general introduction to the construction of medical reality.

This was brought home to me in the context of what was in fact a 'delicate', personal examination rather like Emerson's gynaecological encounter. It occurred in the course of a surgery ward round. We were at the bedside of a man in his thirties who had a swollen and painful testicle. After presenting the case briefly, the consultant asked one of the female students to examine the patient's swollen scrotum. I observed very few bedside teaching sessions in which such examinations of patients' genitals had been involved: I was therefore particularly on the alert for the sort of things that Emerson describes (methods of guarding against embarrassment, repair work when embarrassment occurs and so on). The examination I was observing was 'delicate' in two senses, as it involved a young woman examining a man's genitals, and it was, potentially, extremely painful for the patient and called for careful examination by the student. Immediately after the teaching session I noted:

> I wondered if she would show any embarrassment at examining
> the patient's genitals. She blushed a little, but I could
> detect no other signs of embarrassment on her part.

By the same token I was not able to observe any signs of particular embarrassment, or of affected nonchalance and matter of factness on the part of the patient either. My notes continue:

> Observation, concerning Joan Emerson. She discusses the
> 'clinical' approach as minimising embarrassment. But such
> an approach happens anyway - i.e., in all cases, not only
> in those which involved sexual encounters which might be
> open to misinterpretation. In other words, students will
> generally adopt a 'serious' and 'considerate' approach to
> the patient. It would be difficult to imagine what
> behavioural differences one could expect from situations
> of heightened 'threat'/'embarrassment'....

At this point in my observations, then, I was drawing attention to the fact that Emerson's comments are not confined to gynaecology in their relevance to medical encounters. Rather, they should be seen as describing a special case, throwing into relief features which are general to all doctor patient interactions. In Emerson's terms, the gynaecologist's talk and demeanour can be seen as informing the patient,

'Look, this is a perfectly ordinary clinical encounter - a perfectly normal and routine examination'. But the very fact that it comes over as normal and routine depends upon the fact that this is the nature of all (or most) run of the mill clinical encounters.

The construction of bedside teaching is a variant of 'medical reality management', and we can see how many of the devices that Emerson identifies are mobilised or are available. The medical ambiance does not need construction as a background feature. It is already constituted in the hospital, and patients will already have been socialised into the medical situation by the time they are visited by the clinician and his students. They will at least have been admitted and examined by the resident physician and will have been worked on by the nursing staff. In the same way, there is no need for the explicit recruitment of medical or auxiliary staff to create a medical definition: they are routinely on hand - the houseman performing their day to day duties, the nurses and auxiliary staff theirs.

As part of this process, the medical student's uniform is an important dramaturgical 'prop'. Putting on their white coat is an important symbolic manifestation of students' status passage from preclinical to clinical studies (cf. Becker et al., 1961, p.194). Not only does it symbolise this new status to fellow students, it also declares the wearer of the white coat as a 'medical' person to others in the hospital. For instance, it marks one off from such transients as visitors and out patients, as one strides through the corridors from ward to ward. The white coat may ensure the wearer privileged access in the hospital; it is a passport as one moves about the building.

As a white coated person myself, I was aware of the relative immunity it offered. It provided excellent camouflage as I wandered about, looking for students or their teachers. Indeed, on one occasion, I was rather disconcerted to find that my camouflage had worked too well. Whilst standing with a group of students, waiting for a doctor to teach, I was alarmed to find a member of the public tugging at my sleeve, telling me that a woman had just collapsed nearby, and asking for my help. Luckily I was able to get enthusiastic support from my knot of students; some went for help, whilst others rushed off eagerly to see and join in some real emergency medicine. For the students, too, the white coat confers medical status, and proclaims them as legitimate personnel to the patients and hospital staff. Along with the coat, the student's clinical instruments complete the picture of the young doctor.

The stethoscope, whilst having obvious pragmatic value, is also of great dramaturgical value in proclaiming the clinical student's new found place in the medical hierarchy. During the earliest days in the field, I noticed how stethoscopes were a topic of conversation. Several students pointed out to me how they and their colleagues displayed their stethoscopes as badges of office. Stethoscopes are carried in the roomy pockets of the white coat. But, my informants told me, the more junior clinical students make sure that their instruments are very clearly visible, left dangling artfully over the edge of the pocket, whereas more senior students would stuff their stethoscopes further into their pockets, even out of sight. This, it was suggested to me, may imply that whereas the 'green' fourth year students are eager for clinical work and involvement, their more world weary seniors are as concerned to avoid them. Be that as it may, the

stethoscope, plus the tendon hammer, are obvious emblems of the
students' medical status. By the same token, their possession may
reassure the novitiate and bolster his confidence in the strange new
milieu of the hospital. For instance:

> When we got to the hospital we went to the lockers. The
> students were laughing and joking, rather self consciously,
> I thought, about carrying stethoscopes. One said it was
> because he was hoping to use it soon, and added that it
> also boosted his confidence to be seen carrying it.

To go with their medical 'uniforms' and trappings, further aspects of
the students' self presentation are related to his or her appearance as
a 'medical' person. To some extent, on entering the clinical years,
students are expected to 'smarten themselves up'. During the
preclinical years, the students of the medical school dress much like
any other students. When they go on the wards, some 'standards' may be
imposed.

One senior registrar mentioned to me that he sometimes 'looked twice'
at students, and thought that if he were a patient, he would not fancy
being treated by people who looked like that: but he had never actually
excluded students from the wards on these grounds. There are
'standards' that are normally required throughout all clinical units,
however. These were outlined for some students I was with at an
introductory meeting on the first morning in the hospital:

> Dr Lukes went on to say that some of the students would have
> already visited the wards on a Saturday morning. He added
> that for their work on the wards the men were required to
> wear ties, although suits were not obligatory. Although, he
> explained, the doctors did not insist that men have their
> hair short, he suggested that men with long hair should tuck
> it into the collar of their white coat.

Similarly, in an introductory lecture one physician told the students
that although 'faculty don't care', the patients 'tend to get upset if
people are dressed in a peculiar way or have their hair down to here.
They are to be comforted, not confronted'. It is noticeable that
women's appearance was not specified. The only time when a female
student's personal appearance was commented on occurred while the
students were practising percussing the chest, in the first term on the
wards. The girl in question had long, carefully manicured nails, which
were preventing her percussing properly with the finger tips. The
consultant suggested that she should trim the nails, and I noted that
she had done so by the following morning. Some of the female students
appeared in trousers, but this was never adversely commented on.

There was in fact a wide range of personal styles and modes of dress
current among the students, but observation across the years did suggest
that as they progress through the medical school, they do tend to adopt
more 'sober' and 'conventional', even 'smarter' clothes and hair styles.
This was something which students themselves would sometimes point out
to me, as they directed my attention to their more senior colleagues in
and around the hospitals and the medical quadrangle. Although there
was no miraculous overnight transformation, I did notice how students
began to adopt the style of their senior colleagues. Particularly

during the early days in the field I noticed that the male students would comment on and chaff each other about their clothes and hair styles. Thus, on the first morning of my first year's work, I noted the following interaction in the lecture theatre:

> One student entered in what was clearly a new jacket and tie;
> his hair was fairly long, but well trimmed. He went up to
> sit beside a friend who had shoulder length hair. Seizing it,
> he said, 'This lot will all have to come off'. He then
> turned and pirouetted to show off his own new clothes.

In terms of the students' 'personal front' (Goffman, 1971) this is part of their transformation from laymen to medical men. In parallel with the 'doctrinal conversions' (Davis, 1968) that student professionals go through, they must come to take on the manners (in the broadest sense) of the members of the occupational group. Transformations in self perception are accompanied by transformations in the self that the student presents to others about him, his fellow students, his teachers, and the patients on the wards. At the same time, we can see how this development relates directly to the bedside teaching, insofar as the students' impression management contributes to the successful definition of the situation as a legitimate medical one.

It is not only the students' appearance which is involved here. More generally, their demeanour, and that of the doctors involved, is an important constituent feature of the clinical teaching encounter. 'The bedside manner' is a general, common or garden way of expressing the range of behaviours that are typically expected as distinctive of medical practitioners. While such things are notoriously hard to pin down and document, their general effect is apparent as a background feature of bedside interactions.

Teachers coach students in several aspects of behaviour which are part of the normal demeanour of clinical medicine. An example of this is the injunction that the bed should be approached from the patient's right hand side. The reason for this piece of etiquette is never articulated, but it is often stated as a basic principle of bedside work. Although the requirement may be grounded in practical considerations, it is presented to the students more in the guise of a ceremonial act, rather than one based on convenience of comfort. Sitting on the patient's bed is also a breach of etiquette. It is permissible to perch on it to examine the patient's back; any 'sloppy' sitting on the bed lays a student open to reproof from a clinician.

In much the same vein is the injunction that students should get on the same level as the patient, although here the comfort of the patient is more clearly at issue; students should avoid towering over the patient. Similarly, students are told to make sure that their hands are not too cold when they palpate a patient's body. This can cause further problems, however. On one occasion a student, asked to examine a patient's abdomen, began to rub his hands together, to warm them up. The consultant told him, rather sharply, not to do that - 'It looks as if you're just about to sit down to a good dinner!' Students are also reminded to remake the bed if they have to pull the bedclothes off. This demonstrates consideration for both the patient and the nursing staff.

The observance of such etiquette is one way in which students are coached to respect and reproduce the appearances of medical work. More generally, however, the medical definition of reality requires that some rules of everyday interaction are set aside, and more context specific rules employed. The example of the gynaecological examination, referred to above, is a special case of the demands of such reality maintenance. Clinical work requires that patients' bodies be peered at, probed and felt. Such 'privileged access' is normally confined to intimates, and as Lief and Fox (1963) comment:

> The amounts and occasions of body contact are carefully regulated in all societies, and very much so in ours. Thus, the kind of access to the body of the patient that a physician in our society has is a uniquely privileged one. Even in the course of so called physical examination, the physician is permitted to handle the patient's body in ways otherwise permitted to special intimates, and in the case of procedures such as rectal and vaginal examinations in ways not even permitted to a sexual partner.

Junior students do not normally perform vaginal examinations, though rectals are sometimes done. However, they are routinely expected to perform other sorts of physical examination. Such encounters have to be handled with some care: the participants need to make it clear to one another that this is a 'medical' situation, and not an 'intimate' one. This problem is not entirely confined to the medical arena, but can occur whenever contexts require intimate physical contact (e.g. bodily search by security guards). In all cases the smooth performance of such encounters requires that the actors should treat these events in a matter of fact way. In such interactions - including those involving the medical students - decorum calls for a posture of personal detachment coupled with a display of concern.

For the students, the successful accomplishment of bedside encounters requires that they learn two basic things. First they must manage to treat the occasion as a 'normal', 'medical' one; secondly, they must maintain their composure in a semi public display of their embryonic medical skills. For in their 'on the job' acquisition of competence in bedside work, the students usually have an audience. Inescapably, the patient, if conscious, is in a position to observe their efforts. Frequently, they have to perform with a clinician and their fellow students as an audience as well.

Students frequently encounter difficulties in composure when they first encounter patients on the wards. One student put it quite forcibly:

> It's a terrible experience sort of interviewing patients for the first time....

Other students put it rather less dramatically:

> I've never had any trouble with patients personally....I think I can get on fairly well with most patients. I don't think anybody's ever complained about me....I was very apprehensive. It's a bit worrying as a student to ask people questions about their personal life and

private life, and go into personal problems. You're not
qualified and they know you're not qualified - very
embarrassing to start with.

You have to learn to conquer your initial shyness - that's
the thing I found most difficult - because you feel that
the patient expects so much of you. You know, because, in
their eyes, you're a doctor. And I felt that the first
few sessions I was there I felt it acutely - that they were
very embarrassed for me because I was obviously incompetent.
And that was very difficult at first - and that was one of
the first things we learnt: put on a calm front even
though you haven't a clue what you're doing. The other
thing is to express yourself....

The same girl went on to say,

I don't find it difficult on my own at all; that passed off
pretty quickly. But I still find it difficult to interview
a patient in front of the class. And this is very
difficult, especially if you happen to be landed with a
difficult patient....I really came across my first difficult
patient in front of the class....I asked what was the matter
with her and she, you know, she came back with the classic
reply, 'You should know doctor'. And I was completely
unprepared for it.

   While students can manage to overcome their apprehensions over
interviewing and examining patients, they find their performances
before doctors and their fellow students more nerve racking. As one
student said:

At the ward meetings at the end of the week, they accepted
you as part of the staff. And if you had a patient that
was of interest, you had to present it to the ward, which
was a frightening experience....

And another of the students said,

I don't mind at all having one patient, one person, but I
don't like having surgeons breathing down your neck going
'Tut'.

The presence of clinicians therefore presents the novice student with a
critical audience to their incompetent first trials at clinical work.

   Whilst patients can also be a source of embarrassment to the students,
they may appear to be more indulgent, and students' avowal of their
novitiate status can be employed as a resource. During the early days
of students' time on the wards, they sometimes get lost in their
question and answer sequences, and are forced to consult the small
handbook provided by the medical school:

Dr Saunders said that I could go off with the students if
I liked, and I trotted into the ward, where I found Dennis
Elliott interviewing a middle aged man. Dennis was
referring to his little booklet on 'how to take a history',

and he referred to it several times: as he did so he
apologised to the patient for having to use it.

On such occasions students would offer rather nervous apologies for
having to use this crib, whilst patients would acknowledge that they
didn't mind 'helping' the students. On other occasions, rather more
'covering up' can be employed by the students as they strive to find
their bearings:

> You thought of all the questions to ask and then forgot
> what to ask them next. I would talk about the weather -
> filling in the questions as I started to remember them
> again.

The prospect of a nurse as an audience can also produce fears of
being 'shown up' as incompetent in students as they begin their clinical
work:

> We all met again by the noticeboard. Jeremy Davies and
> David Dean were discussing their respective patients.
> Jeremy had been examining his female patient, and David
> asked him if he had had a nurse present. Jeremy replied
> that he wasn't going to show off his incompetence in
> front of any nurse - he wanted to preserve his 'aura of
> competence'. He asked if a nurse was necessary as a
> chaperone. David thought it wasn't obligatory, but that
> regulations varied from place to place.

Students' inept performances are not always the subject for distress.
On the contrary, the potential problems of their incompetence can be
defused by laughter, and dissolve into general hilarity. For instance,
one student described how humour can arise:

> St.   It'll all come with practice anyway; in the summer
>   when we start clerkships, probably within a week
>   we'll be so good - so used to doing it - that it'll
>   only take a couple of hours. Whereas I can only do
>   the central nervous system in a couple of hours now.
>   Ever seen anybody doing that?
>
> P.A. (untruthfully) No.
>
> St.   You have to try and work out the field of vision, so
>   you hold their head down and get them to look
>   straight into your eye and cover one eye - they have
>   to cover one eye - and then you say 'Tell me when
>   you see my finger', and you turn like that with your
>   finger till they see it moving, and down there till
>   they see it moving...(he demonstrated the tangle that
>   a student can get into)....It's not unknown for the
>   patient to burst out laughing...taking the piss out
>   of the poor student. I think that happened to
>   Loraine Beckett, you know her. Of course she giggles
>   so much anyway. I think when they both got started,
>   the examination ended. Poor Loraine.

The presence of patients as parties to the bedside teaching clearly
constitutes something of a problem for the students in the early days

50

of their clinical work.

INSULATION FROM THE REST OF THE WARD

The scenic and ecological arrangement of bedside teaching emphasises
the two features of clinical education. Insofar as the teaching is
located in a hospital setting, in some respects it does share features
of 'medical' situations. But against that background, the educational
situation is to some extent distinct from the medical milieu. As it
progresses, the teaching round seems almost completed insulated from
the other goings on in the ward. It is, in Goffman's terms, an
'ecological huddle' and as it moves from bed to bed in the ward
enclosed by its 'membrane', to take another of Goffman's terms (Goffman,
1961a).

   As the students cluster round the doctor and the patient's bed they
produce an inward looking gathering, with the patient as the point of
focus. The action is divorced from the rest of the ward about the
group. Frequently the symbolic membrane round the group is given
physical reality as the curtains are drawn round the bed, or screens
brought round to preserve the privacy of the situation, and the doctor
and students crowd round inside the screens. The space round a
patient's bed is usually severely limited - a small territory which
marks the limit on any privacy he can normally claim for himself. The
invasion by a doctor and a group of students (up to twelve in number -
sometimes plus a sociologist) creates a tight scrum, with the patient
in the middle. The patient is entirely enclosed within the group. This
huddle is very rarely intruded upon by the comings and goings of other
people about the ward and the invisible boundary round them is seldom
broken. The students appear on the ward, but they are not of the ward;
they have no clear identity or function within it. Hence there is
little or no call for the students to interact with other medical or
paramedical personnel.

   The hierarchical nature of ward life is also demonstrated in the
separation between the teaching session and the rest of the ward. The
clinician's authority and power ensure routine ward work will not
impinge on his teaching session. During one round I noted:

      at about this point, there was a bit of a commotion as some
      staff (i.e. paramedical staff) were doing something or other
      and chattering rather loudly. Dr McLellan called out
      sharply to them, asking them to be a bit quieter.

As we were inside the screening curtains, I could not see exactly what
was going on beyond the pale. Whether or not the noise was produced
by important clinical work or was idle 'chit chat' I had no way of
knowing. But on an occasion which followed a couple of days later, it
was clear that the disturbance was the outcome of necessary ward work.

      At the nearby bed, porters and nurses were trying to get a
      patient out of bed and onto a trolley: he was very heavily
      built, and appeared to be in a semi conscious state. There
      was a bit of a commotion, as there were four of the nurses
      and a porter trying to do it. Dr Essex stopped teaching
      for a moment, and raised his voice against the noise.

51

'Excuse me do you think you could modify your voice a little?'.

The noise did die down, and the teaching was able to continue. No
explicit reference was made to the patient and what was being done to
him. To some extent, then, the situation parallels that unusual type
described by Goffman (1971, p.33), in which 'the setting follows along
with the performers'. Goffman instances royal processions, funeral
corteges and the like - and the ward round is rather similar to these
paripatetic gatherings. Goffman goes on to suggest that 'In the main,
these exceptions seem to offer some kind of extra protection for
performers who are, or who have momentarily become, highly sacred'. The
degree of sacredness attached to the teaching round depends to a large
extent on the rank of the clinician in charge. The consultant can
generate an aura of inviolable sanctity and exclusiveness, whereas the
more junior grades of staff are less able to produce and sustain such a
definition. In almost all cases, however, the ward round remained set
apart from the rest of the ward.

It is in the nature of the insulation of the students from the rest of
the ward that there is little interaction between them and the nursing
staff. Apart from the occasional informal encounter, I observed next to
no student nurse contact. This is in sharp contrast to popular images
of student activities. It appears to be widely held stereotype that
medical students' work regularly brings them into contact with the
younger members of the nursing staff - to their pleasure - and with the
senior nursing staff - to their chagrin and discomfort. This is, of
course, part of the romantic myth of the general hospital, where nurses
are attractive and sexually available to the male members of staff (cf.
Atkinson, 1971), and which is fostered repeatedly in popular literature,
film and television. It is part of the professional development of the
medical novitiate that he should take on more and more responsibility
for the routine work of the hospital, and to that extent, he comes to
interact more and more with the nursing staff. The students in their
first clinical year do not have such responsibilities, and so they do
not have such working relationships. The lack of contacts between
students and nursing staff was also noted by Becker et al. (1961, p.197)
in their study of Kansas. They also note that popular notions of
medical training tend to overstress the importance of the nurses' role,
and the rate of interaction between students and nurses, and they also
suggest that the idea 'may possibly derive from the very much larger
role she plays in the work lives of interns and residents'.

In the first instance, then, the teaching round is distinct from the
routine work of the wards; it does not enter into the day to day
therapeutic work being performed on the patient. The rounds and bedside
lessons I observed were almost all teaching rounds, conducted by just
one clinician with a group of students. This is in contrast with the
traditional stereotype of the junior students tagging along behind the
consultant and his entourage of registrars and housemen, ward sister
and nurse, occasionally being thrown by a scrap of information as the
consultant checks the progress of his patients. In contrast with this
grandiose and flamboyant picture, the bedside teaching and ward rounds
I observed were generally subdued affairs. The instruction of fourth
year students was, usually, separated from clinician's ward rounds.
Very rarely did nurse or ward sister participate. Again, rarely were
junior students taught along with seniors. On occasions when pressure
of work or staffing shortages meant that teaching and routine ward work

had to be conflated, or where the clinician designated to teach had to perform routine duties, this was taken as an untoward occurrence by the clinicians and an occasion for apologies. For instance:

> Today I went along at 11.15, as the students were doing individual ward work until that time. We then were due to be taught by Dr Harvey: when he arrived he said that we would have to join his ward round, and he was afraid that the juniors would be getting 'a rather raw deal' out of it, and they should butt in and ask questions if there was anything they didn't understand.

The fact that I personally felt uncomfortable in this situation brought home to me the division between the everyday clinical round and the teaching session. Faced with the former I felt an intruder, in contrast to my feeling relatively at home in the latter situation. The continuation of my field notes also underlines the non teaching aspect of the round. Although Dr Harvey, in apologising for the morning's arrangement, had asked the fourth year students to chip in with questions, I recorded after the round:

> In fact there was relatively little questioning on the part of the students, and Dr Harvey did not question them on many occasions.

I am not suggesting that there is necessarily no educational benefit in students' participation in such an exercise, simply that it is not treated as a scheduled part of the teaching programme.

On the other hand, I did record events connected with that ward round which were clearly to do with the day to day clinical work of the ward:

> One old lady had a haematological disorder which was puzzling the physicians. They had ordered a wide variety of tests to be carried out, and the time we spent at her bedside was mainly devoted to the consultant and the junior doctors rifling through the case notes to try to sort out what had been done and what had been discovered.

> Another old lady had been admitted with severe diarrhoea. The houseman wanted Dr Harvey to see her particularly. I could hear the houseman tell Dr Harvey that she had been in the [peripheral] Hospital on a number of occasions but they had been unable to do anything. On Saturday she had been feeling very unwell, very depressed and very much sick and tired of doctors. The hospital had refused to admit her again and her GP had managed to get her admitted to the Royal Infirmary. Dr Harvey looked very cross indeed and snapped, 'In other words, the GP has passed his problem on to us!'

> Whilst this was going on, another houseman came up from the ward downstairs, and told Dr Harvey that a patient had just died. He said something to the effect that their guesses were getting better, and that the patient had died more or less as and when expected. The houseman added that he thought that Dr Jarvis would like to remove some of the organs...: it was necessary to get them fresh, and

they had to be taken in a couple of hours. Dr Harvey said that
if Dr Jarvis would care to arrange that himself, that was
alright - otherwise it could 'go through as normal'. The
houseman said he would 'phone Dr Jarvis, and would also get in
touch with the Medical Superintendent for the permission of the
next of kin.

Such features as these I have reported from my notes did not normally
intrude upon the teaching scene. It was occasionally the case that
clinical duties would compete with a doctor's teaching commitment, but
it was more frequently resolved by the absence of the doctor (e.g.,
called away by his 'bleeper') rather than by a conflation of teaching
and routine work.

The management of the intrusion of such work upon clinical teaching is
also demonstrated by the following extract from my notes:

> Dr Raymond told me, slightly apologetically, that this
> wouldn't be a very formal session, as he would talk about
> some stuff they had been doing last week, and he now wanted
> the students to start thinking about the relative importance
> of the various methods of examining a patient's chest. Also,
> he said, he would be stopping to discuss something with Dr
> Gill [the senior consultant].

He then took his group of students to the bedside of a patient in the
male ward, and set them examining him. My notes continue:

> Whilst the students completed their examination, Dr Raymond
> was talking to Dr Gill and the other members of the chief's
> ward round: I could overhear some of their conversation -
> and could hear that Dr Raymond was telling Dr Gill about the
> same patient as he was teaching on. When he rejoined the
> group of students Dr Raymond had a few words with me,
> telling me that he had to try to strike a balance between
> the needs of teaching and the management of his patients.

I observed something of the same sort of thing in surgical units. On
one occasion, for example, one of the surgeons was due to teach a small
group I had attached myself to. When he came to find us, he explained
rather apologetically that he had routine work to get on with, and this
made his teaching difficult. The problem was that he needed to take
blood from a patient and test the blood gasses on a regular schedule of
half hourly periods, which made it hard for him to give the students
his full attention. In fact he took the students along with him while
he performed the simple procedure and they watched while he did it.
Between blood samples he talked to them about the patient and the test
he was carrying out on her. As a matter of fact, the students seemed
to be quite happy to observe the procedure and follow on while the
surgeon went about his work. This was so to such an extent that when
the clinician returned to the patient at the end of the teaching
session, he clearly expected the students to leave him and wander off;
but he was surprised to find them coming with him once more, to see the
patient again. Although the doctor seemed to assume that the students
would not appreciate this routine work, his assumption was not borne
out. In the event there appeared to be no reason why he should have
apologised to his students. Yet he did so - on the basis that they were

not going to have a specially prepared and laid on teaching session. (Students in fact appreciate such opportunities to 'see things done'). Such 'remedial exchanges' (Goffman, 1972, pp.124 ff.), then, highlight how some varieties of clinical education are normally segregated from the routine work of the hospital ward. This is particularly true of the bulk of 'bedside' teaching; 'apologies' and explanations appear to be appropriate if the two become confused.

The conduct of teaching in the course of on going medical work does occur, in a number of relatively well defined contexts. These are primarily the operating theatre, out patient departments and waiting nights. On such occasions the students are present whilst the doctor works on a patient as part of his normal medical work. Whereas the main preoccupation of the teaching rounds is educational, in these types of encounter the educational tasks must take second place to the diagnostic and therapeutic goals being pursued by the medical staff.

Yet even in these contexts, interaction between students and the hospital staff is minimised. In the out patient clinic, for instance, the location of the consultation within the consulting room or cubicle means that the situation is one which remains confined to the clinician, students and patient. Again, it provides little or no opportunity for the students to engage in routine interaction with hospital personnel outside that focused group. Also, of course, it could be argued that the out patient clinic is itself somewhat removed from the main concerns of the hospital staff and represents a peripheral activity.

In the operating theatre too the students tend to be segregated. By and large they do not participate on the operating theatre floor - and do not therefore interact with the operating team members such as the theatre sister, the scrub nurse, anaesthetist and so on. Either in an open gallery or behind glass they may be spoken to by the operating surgeon, and may be called upon to answer questions on anatomy or surgical technique. But they take little or no active part in the proceedings on the theatre floor: they are observers of the action. But unlike the action the students observe and participate in on the teaching round, at least here the students can observe the 'real' work of the surgical unit rather than specially contrived teaching situations.

Students are least segregated from the routine life of the ward when they attend on waiting nights. As I have already described, the students come into their respective clinical units during the late afternoon or during the evening and can stay well into the night. (How long they do stay depends on their personal interest and motivation, and the amount of action that is going on to hold them there: some nights can be very quiet, others very busy). On these evenings, they are present when new patients are admitted with acute conditions. They therefore have more opportunity to see the work of junior hospital doctors as they admit the patients - take a history and perform a physical examination - and initiate any treatment that is appropriate. On occasion the students may themselves be allowed to take a patient's history. This opportunity to be 'where the action is' represents an important feature in students' perspectives on their clinical instruction and experience.

The point that I have been making is that in some ways clinical teaching is kept distinct from the normal work of the hospital. This can be illustrated further by a consideration of the scheduling and timetabling of clinical work and bedside teaching.

In the first place, a great deal of the work in the wards can be described under the general rubric of <u>routine</u>. The daily round of the patient's life is marked by a recurrent cycle of management by the doctors, nurses and other staff. Although it does not fit Goffman's ideal type exactly, the general hospital displays some features of the 'total institution' (Goffman, 1968). The hospital shares with other institutions of this type the fact that it is an all encompassing organisation. For the inmates (the in patients, that is) the hospital as a complex organisation orders and regulates their life for twenty four hours a day. It is a relatively enclosed community; obviously, it is not so rigidly segregated as a monastery or prison (two varieties that Goffman uses to exemplify the notion) but for the patient in bed, the outside world is not directly accessible, and its representatives (his or her visitors) may only appear for limited periods and at set times. Again, from the patient's point of view, the hospital shares this similarity with the total institution: the fact that to a considerable extent the inmates are 'batch processed'. Although individual patients will have their own regime prescribed for them, and their own pattern of therapy, these individual routines must be set within a wider framework of activity - one in which the patients' daily lives are conducted in lock step. Their lives are collectively scheduled through the ward routine: by the timing of waking up, washing, bedmaking; meals are scheduled; the passage of time is marked by the consultants' and registrars' ward rounds, and so on.

Although they may be less regular in nature, life on the ward is also marked by other types of routine work. The patient's stay may be marked by a timetable of therapy - the collection of urine at regular intervals, the regular removal of blood samples, etc. Similarly, there is a constant background of coming and going by the medical and paramedical staff. Most clearly observable of this is the activity associated with the work of the various specialist units and 'limited practitioners' (Wardwell, 1963) at work in the hospital. Such practice includes that of X-ray departments, physiotherapy, occupational therapy and so on. Indeed, on a busy morning the ward of a teaching hospital is a bit of a bear garden: nurses are busy with their duties; doctors are visiting their patients either alone or in rounds; physiotherapists are walking patients up and down; radiographers wheel portable X-ray machines in and out of the ward; porters wheel patients off to specialist departments for tests, procedures, etc. - and on surgical units they take them back and forth from the operating theatres.

Thus, insofar as there is any observable order, the order of the hospital ward is achieved through the formal and informal coordination of the work of the various specialists and grades of staff; the order is achieved through the ongoing process of negotiation of work practices and their timing (cf. Strauss et al., 1964). Although such order is not always achieved, the smooth running of the ward depends upon the successful interlocking of the various timetables and routines of the various hospital tasks.

In many ways, the <u>teaching</u> which takes place on the wards crosscuts these interwoven patterns of work. Bedside teaching does not necessarily follow the rhythm of the ward. To take a simple example, patients' morning tea or coffee may often lie cold and abandoned on the bedside tables as their elevenses coincide with a visit from the teaching round. Similarly the tail end of the morning's teaching may coincide or overlap with the distribution of the patients' lunches, and so the two activities become mutually disrupting. When the schedules of routine therapeutic work and educational work clash, the entire educational exercise may be threatened. A major consequence of such contingencies is reflected in the problem of <u>access</u> to patients. This becomes particularly crucial for students when allocating to work individually with a patient over several days - to take a full history and complete a full physical examination and hand in a written version plus differential diagnosis. When they come to visit their patient they may quite often find that he or she is unavailable, and is being worked on by other personnel or away in another department.

I frequently spoke with students who were hanging about in the corridors or 'sloping off' for coffee because 'their' patient was not available to answer their questions or submit to their examination.

> I went out to find the students, who were waiting in the corridor. Two or three of them were chatting with one another. Cross said he didn't know how he was going to see his patient this week, as there was an extremely long list of things they wanted to do to him.

As I have indicated, this could arise from a multitude of hospital routines. Students occasionally went into the wards to interview a patient only to find that they were in the line of progress of a ward round led by the chief of the firm, and had to beat a retreat to the canteen or corridor. For students undertaking 'clerking' the problem of access is acute; since they had been allocated to specific patients, the expedient of sidetracking to a different patient or task was not generally open to them. This, of course, contrasts with the position of the teaching physician. He too may find a patient unavailable, but he is able to redefine the work of the session: for instance to discuss the patient *in absentia*, the results of tests carried out on him, present the X-ray pictures. He is also free to move on to another patient, or even to a different illness from the one he originally had in mind.

> Whilst Dr Shepherd was teaching, Dr Mayer came into the teaching room. 'We have a terrible problem', Dr Mayer broke in, 'Mr J. has gone to the [peripheral] Hospital'. Dr Shepherd replied, 'Oh well, he'll be back in a day or two, and the boys can go round and look at him'. (And for the subsequent teaching session, for which the doctors had expected to visit that patient, an alternative topic and a different patient were improvised).

Occasionally, doctors may ignore the disappearance of the patient and conduct the teaching session at the empty bedside. This was sometimes pointed out to me by the students as an extreme example of the 'contrived' nature of some bedside teaching: that such 'clinical' work was done without the participation of the patient. For example:

When we turned to talk to the second patient, we came to an
empty bed, and Mr Jackson explained that, as often happens,
he had been 'whisked away' to X-ray, and that probably his
X-rays had gone with him. Still, he said, he still had the
notes, and we could go back to the teaching room in the
other ward.

   In general, these problems of access involve a postponement of
students' clinical work. However, the competing schedules of therapy
and education may offer more permanent obstacles to the students. Thus
the patient's hospital career may come to an end and all further access
is precluded. Thus, while a student is working on a patient, he or she
may be discharged and sent home:

   Jane Peters had a case history that she had written up, and
   didn't know whom to get hold of to hand it in. John Carter
   had also written up his history but likewise hadn't handed
   it in. Jane Peters said something to the effect that hers
   was the last to get done, and Dougie Callan said that he
   had been unable to complete case notes on his patient, since
   she had gone home. One of the others commiserated on the
   difficulty of having a patient go home.

An alternative outcome, which leads to the cancellation of students'
work rather than postponement, is the death of a patient. Again, as
with the timing of recovery and discharge, the estimated timing of
death is an uncertain eventuality and can be an unforeseen disruption
of the scheduling of educational work.

   Jim Barnes said he hoped that perhaps Dr Roy who was due to
   teach the clinique, might show them the case of paraquat
   poisoning. (The case had received wide publicity in the
   city and was one of a number of similar self poisonings
   that had occurred in recent months). Clay said that the
   patient had died last week. 'How inconsiderate', said
   Barnes.

The two features of the unpredictable timetables of illnesses, and the
divergent schedules of teaching and other hospital work are sharply
highlighted in events which surround the death of a patient.

   Although the patient's death will inevitably interrupt students'
history taking and diagnostic exercises, that patient does not cease to
be an object of clinical and instructional interest. There is the post
mortem to be performed. But the patient may expire at a time which
does not cohere with the schedules of teaching, and the routine of the
pathologists does not necessarily take account of their schedule either.
This can be illustrated from the following case summary.

   The patient in question was an alcoholic, suffering from a
   number of severe problems, including brain damage. He was
   now bleeding from the gut: surgeons had been unable to
   trace the source of the bleeding and further surgery was
   not possible. The patient was barely conscious and it
   appeared that little could be done for him.

   The students examined the patient, and then retired to the

teaching room with the consultant to discuss the management
of the case. At the end of the session the consultant told
the students that this patient would last three weeks,
perhaps less. He would, he added, 'make an interesting post
mortem - you ought to go along'. There were a number of
issues which a post mortem would demonstrate to the students
- one, the exact state of the patient's liver, and, two, the
site and nature of the lesion from which he was bleeding.

Just over a fortnight later, as I chatted with students in
the coffee bar, they were complaining that the patient had
died the night before last, and the post mortem had been
completed the following afternoon, when none of the students
could be present.

The unpredictability of clinical time may also disrupt the smooth flow
of education in surgical units. The teaching of students must be fitted
in with the important work of operating. Whereas physicians may be able
to schedule their rounds with a fair degree of accuracy, surgeons may
find it more difficult to predict the time that they will have to put in
to complete their list of operations. Operations may not prove as
straightforward as first thought, and the time allocated may have to be
exceeded. Once committed to the morning's work in the theatre it must
be completed. Surgeons have less manoeuverability in the possibility
of sidetracking from the schedule of therapeutic work to that of
teaching. Hence students complained that in some units - particularly
those with a small staff complement - they were not infrequently left
stranded with noone to teach them, as the surgeons were unable to get
away from their clinical duties when the timetable indicated.

Thus, in this regard at least, the scheduling of clinical and
educational work presents the students with problems of access both to
patients and to clinical teachers. Indeed Becker et al., (1961)
identify problems of access as the major difficulty facing the Kansas
students in their first clinical year.

The major problem patients present for the student on the
hospital wards, then, is to maintain this continuing
relationship in such a fashion as to be able to get the
necessary information for the job he is assigned. (p.315)

Becker et al. do not cover all the implications of time in the wards.
Hospital wards have a rhythm based upon the patterns of admissions and
discharges. The units admit patients for emergencies on a rota basis,
each ward having a different 'waiting' or receiving night. Thus on,
and immediately after, waiting night, the ward has 'fresh' clinical
material. As the week wears on there will be a diminishing number of
patients for students to see, whose stories have not been told and
examinations taken place.

Thus the turnover of patients in the ward, and the duration of their
stay also have a bearing on the performance of clinical teaching. If
there are many patients in for a lengthy period (e.g. those who are
slowly being rehabilitated after a stroke) then the number of new
patients will be restricted, and units may even run out of fresh
patients to teach on. Such an eventuality may occur in medical units,
but is highly unlikely on surgical wards. The mean duration of

hospital stay varies markedly between general medical and general surgical cases. Available official statistics for the region cite a mean stay of nearly eleven days for surgical patients against eighteen days for medicine. Hence there is a more rapid throughput of patients in surgery, and little danger of fresh clinical problems starting to run out. Thus, to summarise, the dimension of time means that not only do students have problems of access to patients, they also face problems of access to new patients.

As I have indicated in this chapter, then, the nature of the social reality which students encounter is not a straightforward matter. While the rhetoric of clinical experience suggests that the students are immersed in 'real' medicine, we have seen that, like any other medical encounter, bedside teaching must be socially accomplished. Furthermore, the successful management of bedside teaching may even run counter to the social organisation of therapeutic work on the wards. To some extent, as following chapters explore in more detail, the 'reality' of clinical instruction is an artfully contrived version of medical work.

5 The Social Distribution of Bedside Knowledge

This chapter outlines some features of the social organisation of
bedside encounters. Their management rests on the delicate manipulation
of knowledge and information on the part of the doctors and students,
and, on occasion, the patients as well.

THE MANAGEMENT OF AWARENESS AND CONTROL OF INFORMATION

One of the basic constraints that hedges round many hospital encounters
is that involving 'awareness' and information control (see McIntosh,
1974). This has been discussed primarily with regard to dying patients
and their awareness - or otherwise - of their prognosis. Such a concern
is at once a practical one for the doctor and also one that has
generated more theoretical concerns for sociological writing. In the
first instance, the internal debate that a clinician may have to go
through when faced with what he takes to be the knowledge of his
patient's impending death 'to tell or not to tell' is a problem that
confronts the majority of clinicians at some time or other. Secondly,
the grounds on which such decisions are made, and the subsequent doctor-
patient interactions provide an area for the investigation of the
management of professional encounters.

   The most systematic study of the doctor's dilemma and its subsequent
working out is that of Glaser and Strauss (1965). They were
particularly interested in the ways in which social interaction
involving the patient, his relations, nursing and medical staff, is
oriented towards the management of awareness. As their main analytic
framework Glaser and Strauss employ the notion of an 'awareness context'.
They single out four ideal typical awareness contexts - 'open', 'closed',
'suspicion' and 'pretense'.

> An open awareness context obtains when each interactant is aware
> of the other's true identity and his own identity in the eyes of
> the other. A closed awareness context obtains when one
> interactant does not know either the other's identity or the
> other's view of his identity. A suspicion awareness context is
> a modification of the closed one: the interactant suspects the
> true identity of the other or the other's view of his own
> identity, or both. A pretense awareness is a modification of
> the open one: both interactants are fully aware but pretend not
> to be.   (Glaser and Strauss, 1964)

In the course of their hospital ethnography, Glaser and Strauss trace
the interactions whereby such contexts are constituted, maintained or
transformed. For instance, they examine the coalitions and teamwork
whereby physicians and nurses work together to keep a patient they
believe to be dying in a state of ignorance about their prognosis.

   The adjudication of the gravity of medical news, and its possible effects on the patient (whether or not the physicians have pronounced him to be 'dying') is an ever present feature of bedside teaching and clinical work. At the outset of their work on the wards students are explicitly coached in the need to maintain awareness contexts: this is especially crucial in the case of closed awareness. On the first day in the hospital with a group (it was their first day on the wards too) we had an introductory talk which included the specific injunction that students should 'exercise extreme care at the patient's bedside, and put oneself in the patient's place. One does not talk about cancer, carcinoma, tumour, syphilis....' And on the following day, during one of the introductory lectures, I made the following notes:

> Avoid use of word 'cancer', although you may use it in reassuring the patient that he hasn't got it....

> With the recent publicity on the harmful effects of smoking, it is now very important how you frame your questions about smoking. Patients will leap to the conclusion that you suspect cancer....

Beyond such maxims and advice, the students I observed at Edinburgh did not receive more formal injunctions on the topic of awareness closure. But at another Scottish University, the students receive such explicit instructions as part of their introductory hand-out for the clinical course ('Notes on the Examination of Patients'). At the foot of the first page, these instructions include:

> A warning: When discussing medical matters in the patient's hearing, certain words with disturbing associations should be avoided. This is so even if they are not relevant to the particular individual. Such words with alternative euphemisms are -

Malignant disease, cancer growth	- neoplasia or new tissue formation
Syphilis	- specific disease or lues
Gonorrhoea	- Neisserian infection
Post-mortem	- Sectio cadaveris, the Professor of Pathology's wards
Death	- Exitus

> Each clinician has his own method of periphrasis and especially in front of intelligent patients some obliquity of expression is to be commended.

The use of such periphasis and synonymy was frequently recorded in my field notes - although I did not encounter the exotic 'Professor of Pathology's wards'. Clinicians and students alike used terminology such as 'space occupying lesions' for tumours, and 'neoplasia' or 'neoplastic process' for 'cancer'. (Students complain that such periphrasis is becoming hard to sustain. The wide dissemination of information about disease processes - particularly malignancy - in recent years makes it difficult to ensure that an alternative word or phrase is unknown to the patient. Not only has 'carcinoma' joined 'cancer' as a lay term (and hence become unusable), 'neoplasia' is also becoming too familiar a term for comfortable use at the bedside).

John explained that they were always warned against the use of
emotive terms in front of the patient. You don't say lung
cancer or use common terms like angina. Instead of cancer you
say something like 'the lesion may be mitotic in origin'. He
also said that the word 'neoplasm' was getting too well known
by the public.

Teaching presents a possible threat to the preservation of closed
awareness contexts that have been negotiated by the hospital staff vis-
a-vis their patients. This is so on two counts. First - and in the
early days of the year this was especially so - students may unwittingly
blurt out medical information which the clinician may wish to remain
covert. Secondly, while students and staff may be aware of the
necessity for awareness management, and students may orient their talk
towards such a consideration, the very nature of teaching places great
strain on the preservation of closed contexts. The act of teaching must
make accountable for the participants (the students in particular) the
basic features of the patient's history. As such accounting must be
done publicly, talk may be open to the scrutiny of the patient in a way
which does not normally occur. There is less possibility of the doctor
making some brief, muttered comment and passing on. If he wishes to
spend any time at all in using a patient as a teaching resource, then
the interaction at the bedside is always liable to render the accounting
of his illness open to the patient, and thus to threaten previously
negotiated contexts. Templeton (1964) touches on this point in his
observations on bedside teaching:

> ...the reporting of the patient's history and physical findings
> at the bedside placed the student in a paradoxical position of
> trying to choose vocabulary that would both clearly explain the
> problem to the group but which of necessity would keep certain
> facts from the patient...and discussions which took place in
> the patient's presence without including the patient as a
> participant inevitably exposed the patient to...unpleasant
> focus on the unfavourable aspects of the patient's prognosis.

Thus, the accountability of the illness and the patient's potential
access to knowledge of his condition as it is made public, may provide
grounds for the patient moving from a state of closed awareness to one
of suspicion. Students can therefore find themselves confronted by the
problem of how to discuss things with their teachers without spoiling
the patient's state of awareness, or causing distress. As one student
put it,

> 'When you're asked to discuss what you think is wrong with the
> patient...I wish we could go away from the earshot of the
> patient....You might say the wrong thing. You think
> desperately how you can describe the lump without frightening
> people....'

Hospital patients have been observed to try to elicit information from
various types of personnel in the wards. The patient who is anxious or
suspicious as to the nature of his or her condition will attempt to
'pump' people for information. If doctors will not divulge what the
patient feels to be sufficient information then the nurses will be
turned to (Glaser and Strauss, 1965, p.55 ff.). The students who come
to talk to them also offer patients a further possible source of
knowledge. Hence it is a continuing concern of students to guard

against divulging information. Several of the students I interviewed told me that when they were clerking a patient individually they had been asked 'awkward questions'. To quote just one:

> Heather Morgan had had a patient ask her about her condition
> on her first day of clinical work in medicine. She added
> that she had had to 'hedge' and avoid giving the patient a
> direct reply.

Glaser and Strauss describe how the nurses were able to avoid such problems, to some extent at least, by referring patients to the chain of command on the ward. They were able to deflect unwelcome or embarrassing questions by telling the patients that they should ask the doctors about their condition and prognosis. As the authors quote, they would use a variant of the reply 'I don't know, I'm not a doctor'. In precisely the same way, the students can employ their novitiate status as a resource in resolving any potentially difficult or distressing 'suspicion context':

> If patients do ask awkward questions about their condition,
> then it is an easy let out to say that you are a student,
> and to tell the patient to ask one of the senior physicians
> about it.

Thus the students can claim either that it is not their place to discuss such things with the patients, or that, by virtue of their ignorance, they are not in any position to do so anyway.

A problem in this regard arises from the students' infrequent and spasmodic contact with any given patient. Since they have not normally followed a case from admission to the ward, through the remainder of the patient's hospital career, students are not always in a position to tell what the patient knows or does not know already. Hence it may be particularly problematic for them to judge what to impart to the patient about his illness, since they are not 'clued in' to the previous negotiations between staff members and the patient in question.

> Heather told me that two of them had been talking to a
> patient who had asked them about her condition. The
> students hadn't known how much she knew already, and so
> had no idea how much they could reasonably tell her.

The students' dilemma in this matter is made worse since different clinicians employ different 'rules of thumb' in deciding how much information to divulge to patients. As one student put it, 'some consultants are adamant that the patient should never be told; others believe that it depends on the patient concerned'.

When patients use the students as an alternative source of information they are sometimes successful in eliciting reassurance. It is by no means unheard of for patients to imagine that they are much more gravely ill than is the case, and if they voice their fears, then students can try to put their minds at rest. When illness is not serious or terminal, then students are at liberty to offer information and explanations. One of the students, Alan Pickering told me that -

> A patient he was clerking had come in after a bleed: the

patient thought he was still bleeding, as he was passing black
stools. He was worried, but was unwilling to talk to the
doctors about his fears. Alan was able to reassure him that
the colour of his motions was caused by the iron tablets that
he was now taking.

When the doctors appear unapproachable, more junior personnel are turned
to by patients (cf. Cartwright, 1964). A concern for the management of
information is therefore something which students must learn in
accomplishing medical encounters.   There are, however, occasions on
which it is the patients who must take care over divulging information
in the course of bedside teaching. This is particularly so in the case
of patients who are relatively 'well-informed' about their own condition.

THE WELL-INFORMED PATIENT

Many patients in the teaching hospital have control over a vital
resource in the bedside teaching encounter: that is, a degree of
knowledge and understanding of the diagnosis and treatment of their own
illness. Such information can derive from a number of different
sources, as can be illustrated at the outset from the following
fieldnote extracts; they were written while I accompanied a male
student who was 'clerking' a patient, a middle aged woman.

Pt.   I pass too little water - compared with other people
       that is...they give you a 24 hour collection and you
       notice that there's nothing there compared with
       other people.

St.   What are the water tablets you take?

Pt.   Lasex
       ....

St.   What medicines were you on before you came into
       hospital?

Pt.   Lasex and Ponderax. The chemist told me they were
       the most expensive pills around.
       ....

The student asked if there was anything else in her
previous history. The patient replied that she had been
'in surgical' - 'I had a lipoma on the chest'.

The student asked the patient about her obstetrical
history - 'Were they delivered normally? You weren't
cut open?'

Patient: No it wasn't a caesarean.
....

St.   Any diabetes?

Pt.   No, not according to the tests - they've found
       something now - I'll not tell you.

St.   I'll look it up in the files.

Pt.   That's no good - they don't know what it is. I
       was going home on Saturday.

From this simple sequence of student-patient interactions we can identify a number of possible sources of information which go together to form her history. They are: observation and comparison with other patients; interaction with the pharmacist; her previous hospital visits; her previous interactions with clinicians in the course of her present hospital stay. Thus from her previous visit she can refer to her lipoma and from her current visit admission she can herself report on the negative results of tests for diabetes mellitus. Although she cannot offer the student any definitive results, she can alert him to the fact that further tests have been undertaken and their results noted by the clinician.

Clearly, the range of knowledge available to the patient, the detail, the degree to which it is warrantable by reference to medical opinion and theory - these will all differ from individual to individual. Yet we can begin by sketching in some of the relevant features which are implicated in the process of sharing and gaining medical information.

An example of a patient's understanding which stemmed from a long medical history and a close relationship with the medical profession is provided below:

> At 11.15 Dr Lewis came in to take us to a patient. She took the whole group (12 students and myself) to the women's ward ....We all gathered round a patient's bedside, and Dr Lewis asked one of the men to begin taking her history....

> The student began by asking the patient what had brought her into hospital, and Dr Lewis broke in to tell him that it was not the present complaint that was of interest. The student therefore asked the patient to tell him about her medical history. (It was largely inaudible to all but those immediately by the patient's head, and I could see those at the back of the group craning their necks and straining to distinguish what was going on. All I could catch at this stage was that the patient had suffered a haemorrhage after the birth of her daughter).

> After a minute or two Dr Lewis asked the first student to summarise the history, and suggested that a diagnosis was possible at this stage.

> The student summarised his findings - including the original haemorrhage, a history of sluggishness, and poor tolerance of cold. When the student mentioned that Mrs G. had had poor tolerance of cold weather, Dr Lewis butted in and asked 'Did she tell you that?' 'Yes', he replied. Dr Lewis turned to the patient and said that she mustn't 'give anything away'. Mrs G. agreed not to, with a cheerful, rather conspiratorial expression.

> The student stated that he thought that the patient had Simond's disease, and this was confirmed by Dr Lewis. From then on, Dr Lewis conducted the group session almost entirely alone, with some participation from the patient, and just one or two contributions from individual students.

> Dr Lewis told the group that the patient had a long history, and that she had first seen her when she herself was an SHO.

She described to the students how rudimentary treatment was when at the time she first saw Mrs G. Dr Lewis said that Mrs G. was one of the 'Edinburgh collection' suffering from Simmonds disease with various degrees of severity.

The patient herself commented on her comatose condition in cold weather, and referred to it as her 'hibernating'. Dr Lewis seized on this image as a particularly apt one to describe a common characteristic among sufferers from Simmond's disease.

Dr Lewis talked about the possible treatment of the disease and asked the students how they would set about it. One of the students suggested hormone therapy, and Dr Lewis said at one time they had treated Mrs G. with doses of ACTH. At the time it had been very difficult to estimate dosages with any accuracy, and the treatment had been very difficult and uncertain. At this point the doctor and her patient engaged in a private reminiscence about their early treatment and its tribulations. The patient exclaimed that, despite all the difficulties, 'Oh, it was worth it...it made such a difference'.

As Dr Lewis was leading up to the discussion of the ACTH therapy, the patient kept looking up at her, smiling and winking. I got the impression that they were sharing a more or less private joke about the vicissitudes of that treatment and its hazards.

The interaction between Dr Lewis and her patient was, throughout the half hour or so that we were at the bedside, very much a private relationship, going on with shared memories. The students took very little part in these proceedings.

The patient's own career spanned a number of years, and had developed in parallel with the doctor's professional career; she had been in on the early development of hormone therapy, and could trace its subsequent implementation from her personal experience. She had enjoyed a status which closely paralleled that described by Fox (1959). Thus the dynamics of the teaching session were affected by the closely cooperative relationship that had grown up between doctor and patient over a number of years. Having gone through her own 'experiment perilous', she had become extremely well informed on Simond's disease - its aetiology, symptoms and treatment. She appeared to take considerable pride in her position as a 'well-informed patient' and her privileged status as a long standing 'guinea pig' who had participated in the Edinburgh work on hypopituitarism.

On more than one occasion, the knowledge possessed by 'well-informed patients' outstripped that of the fourth year students themselves. Such superior knowledge on mastery of technical vocabulary on the part of patients may threaten the students with a loss of face. It may be felt to undermine their position as medical men and women. Just as it was a great talking point whether patients had called a student 'doctor' or not, this self perception of 'young doctor' could be a precarious one. Sustained by the student's successful production of appropriate demeanour and expertise, it can be undermined by a failure of medical understanding on their part.

Insofar as the patient's fluency with medical terminology and information can threaten the students' position, they may be led to discount the patient's competence. Patients were sometimes implicitly accused of using such medical vocabulary without necessarily understanding it. For example, during the early weeks of the year, the students I was with practised taking psychiatric and social histories from patients in the general medical wards. Having done so, they then presented their case histories to the rest of the clinique and a lecturer in psychiatry. In presenting a report on 'their' patient, two of the students repeated sections of her history verbatim. It appeared that she was using a wide range of semi-technical and medical vocabulary. The psychiatrist brought this to the students' attention as a possibly significant feature of the patient's general attitude:

> The lecturer suggested that Mrs J. liked to be very informed on the use of medical terms - she had been able to name the drugs she had been on, had used terms like 'debility' and so on. Doug Ewart replied, 'I wouldn't say she was <u>informed</u>, but she liked to use the words'.

Here perhaps the lecturer appeared more willing to credit the patient with a degree of well-informedness. The students on the other hand, seemed less keen to credit the patient with any genuinely useful information. On the basis of the history as the students presented it, there were no external criteria to judge whether the patient was presenting the information accurately. The doctor was willing to give her the benefit of the doubt, the students were not.

In comparison with the general lay population or patients visiting clinics, the patients in a teaching hospital who cooperate in the teaching of clinical subjects are in a better position to develop a well-informed perspective on their illness. Patients who have come to be defined as 'interesting' cases for the purposes of instruction may be visited by doctors and students on numerous occasions. They are not only required to reproduce their history time after time but may also listen to bedside discussions of their condition. Such instructional discussion provides a good opportunity for patients to glean knowledge of their own case.

PATIENTS AS LEGITIMATORS AND COACHES

I have already described how the patients may be seen by students as threatening their display of medical competence. If well-informed patients appear to know more than the students themselves, then it becomes difficult for the students to sustain a convincing performance as legitimate medical people. Their novitiate status and relative ignorance will be 'shown up' by the patients. By the same token patients can legitimate students' performances. Not only can patients provide students with a general legitimation of their role as doctors in the making, they can also provide more detailed legitimation of students' performance of their work. (That is, quite irrespective of whether they see them as 'students' or 'doctors', the patients can openly acknowledge the successful accomplishment of clinical tasks). Given the patients' position as team members in sustaining the reality of the bedside session, they may be in a position to comment on the teaching session and the members' competence.

In one session I observed the students were examining a middle aged woman. They had been informed explicitly by the consultant that they were to examine 'these neurological legs'. There was thus no question of secrecy vis-a-vis the patient, and the patient appeared to be well aware of her condition. As the examination progressed, one of the students tried to elicit <u>clonus</u> (a form of reflex) but was unable to do so. The consultant then demonstrated his own technique, and successfully elicited the sign. The student tried again, using the consultant's method - he produced <u>clonus</u> for himself this time, and the patient, nodding and smiling announced to the world at large, 'He's got it!'

Or again:

Cons. You asked him (an elderly male patient) about his eyes
       ...you asked a very general question and got an answer
       about visual acuity...but there's one thing you must
       ask....

St.   (to patient) Did you ever get double vision?

Pt.   No...turns to consultant...was that the question?

Cons. Yes.

The patient turns back to the student, grins and makes a thumbs up sign to him.

In addition to such unsolicited, spontaneous interventions from the patient, it also remains possible for the teaching clinician to acknowledge the position of the patient, and to use him or her to evaluate a student's examination or diagnosis. This strategy can be seen at work in the course of the following extract from my field notes. I reproduce it quite fully as it also demonstrates a clear case of a patient with a fairly full and detailed knowledge of her own (complex) medical history.

Dr Rosen asked what had originally been wrong with the patient. She replied, 'I had a gall bladder'.

Dr Rosen replied good humouredly, 'We all have a gall bladder'.

Mrs B corrected herself, 'I had a gall bladder removed I mean'.
....

Dr Rosen continued, 'Was the operation a success or not?'

'Just before the end of the operation I passed out, and that was me out for three days'.

Dr Rosen explained, 'As I understand it from reading the notes, she went into deep shock and needed resuscitation for three days'.

There then followed a lengthy technical discussion between the physician and the students on the possible causes of the patient's collapse. This was followed by a discussion of the biochemistry of the patient's present disorder. Dr Rosen asked, 'What disease is that?'

A student replied, 'Addison's disease'.

Dr Rosen turned to the patient, 'Is that right?'

'That's right', the patient confirmed.

Dr Rosen asked Mrs W. 'Would you like to tell them what you had then and have been taking since?'

'Cortisone, thirty seven and a half a day, and....'

Dr Rosen interrupted and stopped her saying any more about the details of the therapy, saying he would go into that later.
....

Dr Rosen went out of the ward for a minute or two, and the students chatted to the patient. One of them asked her if she had two specific symptoms of Addison's disease. She told them that she had not. 'That is what is so puzzling about me - I haven't got all the right things, or they're all upside down....I'm sorry I've landed you with all this'.

'It's all part of our education', said Tim Watson.

In terms of her knowledge of her previous history and therapy this patient comes over as very well informed indeed. In fact, given the 'puzzling' nature of her case, she appeared to know almost as much about it as her doctors did - or at least as much as they could be sure of. As the doctor himself indicated, her previous history is not clear, and again, she seems to know as much about it as can be seen from the official record of her previous operation in the case notes available. It seems therefore entirely in keeping with the picture of the distribution of knowledge that emerges here that the consultant in charge should explicitly turn to this patient and invite her to act as adjudicator of the students' diagnosis of her condition - something which is normally done only by the doctor.

In a similar way the patients, as participants in the teaching situation, may be in a position to 'clue in' the students. They may be able to coach the students in their clinical performances. They can indicate what it is that 'the doctors normally do', and direct the students towards relevant clinical approaches. Hitherto I have discussed patients' cooperation in sustaining the bedside situation in terms of their acquiescing to a more passive role: in supporting 'cold' medicine, the patients are normally required to act in a 'passive' way - their cooperation lies in not intervening to provide clues to the student. However, from their vantage point of 'inside knowledge' the patients can intervene in a more active way to direct the students' endeavours.

This can be illustrated in the following field note extracts, where patients concerned volunteer information to the student in an attempt to establish a successful encounter with them.

I followed John up to the female ward...and joined him at the bedside of a woman, who was sitting in her armchair, wrapped in a dressing gown. She looked slightly exasperated as we walked through the curtains. John stopped and looked through his notebook. 'I must make sure which eye I'm supposed to be looking in'. The patient, with an air of exasperation, replied, 'It's my right eye. I thought all this was finished'.

Edwards and Bell both looked at Mrs C's eyes. 'They normally do that with the light thing', she told them. (Presumably referring to an opthalmoscope).

The same phenomenon has been noted by Stokes (1974:24-5) writing on 'the clinical examination',

> There is...a need to look more closely at the type of patient who is pressed into service for the examination. Too often there have been 'professionals' who have made themselves available to hard pressed registrars entrusted with the organisation of the examination. Considering the central role they play, their financial remuneration is, in general, paltry, so they cannot do it for the money; it is probably the power which attracts them, the opportunity to suppress a vital piece of history, occlude a physical sign and so influence a candidate's chance of passing; this may occur at a subconscious level and the most chronic professional patients like to constitute themselves as assistant examiners (some of them have become quite skilled).

A number of the patients that students see, then, are well informed and they have control over important resources in the teaching situation. Likewise the chances are that the doctor will also have knowledge of what has already been done to the patient. These are provided for by the organisation of 'cold' medicine. But if that exercise is to come off successfully then it must pass as simulating 'hot' medicine. Despite the fact that the diagnosis and therapy may already have been undertaken the student's practice should proceed as if this were not the case. Thus in producing the distinctive status of the reality like bedside teaching session such previously accumulated knowledge must be managed with care. If the patient should blurt out the diagnosis applied to his or her trouble, then the reality like features of the exercise will be largely nullified.

It is therefore a concern in the construction of such encounters that patients and doctors should be engaged in monitoring the flow of information. They need to attend to what may be told and when. This concern can be illustrated by the following field note extract.

> The students had been told to examine the patient's precordium, one by one. As the first student began, the registrar came back and poked his head through the curtains to see if everything was OK.
>
> Pt. 'Doctor, do I tell them what's wrong?'
>
> Dr. 'Under no circumstances....If they ask you what's wrong, ask them their names and I'll come back and find out who they are'.
>
> Pt. 'It's just that the other day I was told not to tell them, but I slipped....'.

The following extract also illustrates the point:

> A girl student was exploring whether the patient (an elderly lady) had any signs of anaemia. As she was examining her eyes, the inside of her mouth, the creases in her palms, etc.,

the old lady chipped in 'I've had a blood transfusion since I came in....'

The doctor interrupted, 'Don't tell them too much...you're giving the whole show away...giving away the whole shooting match!'

The old lady clapped a hand to her mouth.

These two extracts clearly illustrate how patients and doctors can jointly engage in monitoring and controlling the transmission of knowledge between themselves and the students. Such a joint production serves to ensure that the students' diagnostic work should adequately parallel the processes of 'real' medicine. The encounter is treated in such a way as to reproduce the ways in which the inquiry should proceed - as if the diagnosis had not in fact already been done. In this way 'cold' medicine can be done in such a way as to mimic the nature of 'hot' medical work.

The following field note extract shows clearly how the consultant can set about controlling the use of previously acquired information. In this instance, the doctor established a 'meta-game', which provided the rationale for following the rules of cold medicine teaching. Jokingly, he provided a setting for an interaction in which the patient's own resources of information could be held in abeyance.

The consultant began the teaching session by telling the students, 'Imagine that Mr_____ is an Eskimo, who's deaf and dumb and mentally deficient...; in other words they were not to take a history, but were to proceed straight to a physical examination. As the various students took the patient's pulse, examined him for sacral oedema, tested his eye movements, examined his thyroid, etc., the consultant commented to the patient that he was 'doing fine', and that he was using him as a 'male model'.

The consultant then asked one of the students to examine the patient's precordium. When the student opened the patient's pyjama jacket, he exposed an old operation scar on the left side of the man's chest.

Pt.   'Do I tell them about that?'

Cons. 'No...as far as they're concerned that's a shark's tooth that tore you apart....'

In this extract we can detect some of the features of the distribution of knowledge. Hitherto in the session (which I have severely edited) the knowledge and information which was being used in the teaching session had been entirely the prerogative of the consultant. Now, as his scar was exposed, the patient's personal knowledge was brought into play, and his ability to divulge or keep back this information became a crucial resource in the teaching interaction. The consultant brought the patient back into line by reaffirming his fictional role and so re-established his 'conspiracy of silence' with the patient.

The following extract also exemplifies how physicians may orient their teaching practices to the possibility of the patient divulging the diagnosis to the students before the students themselves have gone through the history and attempted their own differential diagnosis.

> The first patient that Dr Porter took us to see was a lady in
> her seventies...Dr Porter asked her if we could look at her
> tummy. She pulled up her nightdress to reveal a band of sore
> places round her midriff.

> Dr Porter asked Bell, 'What do you think that is?', and
> turning to the patient added, 'Don't tell them what it is'.
> Bell looked at her in silence for some moments, then said,
> 'She might as well tell me what it is....'

> Dr Porter hinted, 'Remember - the accent is on neurology'.

> 'Herpes zoster', volunteered one of the other students.

> 'Herpes zoster', repeated Dr Porter approvingly.

It must be emphasised that under conditions of 'cold' medicine, the
teaching doctor will normally be well informed about the patient. He
himself will have seen the patient before, or will have access to the
accumulated knowledge about the patient, through discussion with
colleagues, clinical conferences, and the folder of case notes. By
virtue of such resources he can guide the students' history taking and
diagnoses - and guide the patient as well, if need be. This aspect of
the teaching situation can be demonstrated from the following transcript
excerpt. One of the students had been told to take a history from the
patient. After a few minutes of question and answer between him and the
patient, the consultant broke in:

> 'Okay, fair enough. Now I would like you, in turn, to ask
> relevant questions - one question each - trying to get
> further into his history. And I think it is only fair to
> say that so far you have not elicited all the main symptoms.
> What other questions are you going to ask?'

Here we can see how the previously accomplished diagnostic work
informs these comments. The consultant's advice that there is still a
symptom to be drawn from the patient implies that there is some already
established list of symptoms. This is available as a topic for the
physician by virtue of the fact that he himself has already taken a
history, or has a history available in the folder of case notes. Here
the consultant's guiding hand was needed further, as the students'
history taking continued. Despite the fact that the consultant had
offered his intervention, that elusive further symptom was not
forthcoming. The consultant therefore turned to prompting the patient:

St.	'Is there anything else that you feel - symptoms that you get with the pain?'
Pt.	'No, it's just the pain I feel. That's all, nothing else'.
Cons.	'Is that actually strictly true? You know, is there anything - I think the question really is - is there anything which is happening recently?'
Pt.	'Well, apart from the pain I seem to have been drinking, lots of water, milk, things like that. Because of this, I seem to go to the toilet a lot

more than I used to....'

Here the physician orients the patient to the possibility that there
may be another symptom - that there is additional information that they
are both aware of. The consultant now indicates that this item of
information may now be legitimately divulged by the patient to the
students. Again, his ability to do so rests on the 'cold' nature of the
teaching exercise. The doctor can overcome the patient's lack of
forthcomingness because he is well aware of this symptom <u>and</u> he knows
how it can be elicited. He reformulates the student's question in such
a way that it will elicit the symptom that he is hoping will be elicited.
He does this by introducing the notion that things that have been
happening to the patient <u>recently</u> are what is really at stake (whereas
the student's own question gave no indication of recent symptoms -
indeed, it could not possess the necessary knowledge needed to formulate
it in this way).

What we have seen in the above extracts, and in the previous
discussion of well-informed patients, shows how the teaching clinician
can manage the situation. By virtue of his knowledge of the patient and
his illness, he can 'orchestrate' the flow of information between the
patient and his students. He can help to create the 'reality like'
features of the academic exercise by ensuring that knowledge is
suppressed when necessary; he can also create the opportunities for
information to be divulged when it is appropriate. He is engaged in
'meta-communication' - that is, talk about talk. Stubbs (1975) has
argued that meta-communication is a particularly important feature of
teachers' talk. Teachers are constantly engaged in monitoring who can
talk, for how long, to whom and about what (and in schools, the level of
noise). In the case of the teacher at the bedside, he is engaged in
talking about the talk of the other parties. He too is concerned to
monitor who is talking (patient or student; which of the students) and
the content of their talk. His meta-communication is oriented towards
ensuring the orderly exchange of information between the other two
parties in the course of the triadic interaction at the bedside.

Here again the patient in the next extract from my notes, begins to
give 'the game' away, as he starts to divulge to the students a crucial
piece of information that the consultant apparently wants to save until
later in the interaction. The patient in question was an elderly man
whom the students were questioning in connection with what appeared to
be symptoms of neurological impairment.

    Dennis continued, 'Do you ever have ringing in the ears?' Dr
    Porter looked approvingly at him. The patient replied, 'No,
    but when the doctors use what I'd call a tuning fork....' Dr
    Porter broke in, 'You're giving away all the trade secrets'.

What the patient was referring to was indeed a tuning fork, which is
normally used in neurology to test for patients' sense of vibration. It
is struck and placed on some bony part of the body (e.g. the ankle
bone). Later in the same situation, the physician was getting the
students to say what they would want to test the patient for, and to
perform these neurological tests.

    Dr Porter asked, 'What else?' There was a period of silence,
    as none of the students volunteered a reply. Finally he

reached behind the head of the bed and produced a large tuning
fork. 'Vibration' chorused some of the students.

If we return to the nature of 'cold' medicine, we can begin to amplify
the material I have just discussed. 'Cold' medicine is an opportunity
for the students to practise the techniques of clinical method.
Although both the patient and the doctor may know the nature of the
patient's illness, such knowledge has to be set aside for the purposes
of the teaching exercise. By acting 'as if' previous clinical work had
not been done, and knowledge not accumulated, the members of the
clinique, the doctor and the patient, can re-enact a scene which
displays features of 'hot' medicine. The teaching session can be
conducted by the clinician in charge in such a way as to parallel the
routine of history taking etc., as it is done on 'fresh' patients in the
acute phase of their conditions. Thus, although the patient may be
aware of the nature of his illness, or of critical features of his
hospital career, the successful accomplishment of the situation demands
that the shared knowledge enjoyed by the patient and the doctor should
be temporarily suppressed, until it is methodically uncovered by the
students in the course of their investigations.

THE DOCTOR'S PRIOR KNOWLEDGE

The doctor's prior knowledge of the patient's condition means that he is
often in a position to produce displays of skill and competence in
clinical technique. That is, over and above the fact that the doctors
enjoy superior expertise in general, they also have a particular
advantage in relation to the patient they are teaching on. If they
already know what they may expect to find - especially when performing a
physical examination - then they are in an advantageous position to
bring off an impressive display of clinical acumen and skill. This is
particularly so if they have previously examined the patient and then
can simply rehearse what has been done already, and can 'work back' from
the predicted result. This is, I think, illustrated in the following
extracts of field notes, which were taken from the same teaching session
(in medicine). The students involved were examining an old man who had
given them a history of dizziness, loss of balance and double vision;
they were performing a series of tests on the central nervous system.

Dr Porter asked the students what further tests can be used
for proprioception. Grant suggested the Romberg test. Dr
Porter asked him to describe it. Grant described how one
gets the patient to stand upright, with the eyes shut; they
lose their balance, he explained, as they are normally using
visual stimuli to maintain their balance. Dr Porter asked
how one might reproduce the Romberg test in the upper limbs.
Jackson suggested getting the patient to touch the tip of
his nose with his eyes shut. Dr Porter pointed out that the
Romberg test does not involve movement. He himself (as no
further suggestions were forthcoming) asked Mr F. to hold
his arms straight out in front of him and shut his eyes. The
patient did so, and Dr Porter exhorted him to 'Keep them
there...keep them there...', but gradually his left hand
started to waver, and though his right hand remained steady,
the left hand slowly drooped. Dr Porter looked round
triumphantly, 'I'd like a round of applause for that!'

Later in the same encounter:

> Dr Porter then tested for the possibility of the patient
> ignoring one side of his body. The doctor got him to close
> his eyes and say which arm he was touching, the patient
> successfully identified which one it was, but when both arms
> were touched simultaneously, he only reported feeling his
> <u>right</u> arm being touched. 'I trust you're all impressed',
> commented Dr Porter.

Here the doctor had taken the initiative in conducting the examination.
The students, despite questioning from the doctor had not suggested the
best and most appropriate tests of neurological functioning. Hence, the
consultant had had to introduce the tests off his own bat. His tests
were totally successful - quite 'dramatically' so (cf. his call for
applause). Although he would probably have performed these tests
anyway, given his neurological expertise, on the basis of the history as
presented, the success of his demonstration was pretty well guaranteed
for him by virtue of the previous work that he and his colleagues had
performed with this particular patient.

The clinical tests for neurological functioning lend themselves
particularly to such 'dramatic' performances. The patient who
involuntarily acts out the signs of his impairment appears as the
physician's unwitting 'stooge' in his demonstration of clinical
expertise. In the course of one neurology session I noted that the
consultant referred several times to his getting the patient to do her
'party tricks', and spoke of his having 'trained' her to do them
properly (which is itself a further acknowledgement of the clinical
teacher's previously acquired information). However, although the
doctor is in this advantageous position to adopt such a thaumaturgical
approach, this does not necessarily mean that he will always be able to
bring them off successfully. The doctors' performances occasionally
fell very flat indeed, if the patient failed to respond as predicted.

> Dr Fowler began to speak to the patient, and told us to watch
> her closely. (The patient - an old lady - was fairly drowsy
> and didn't appear to be altogether 'with it'). As he spoke
> to the patient, he gestured to Heather Muir to sidle right up
> to the end of the bed - so that she was next to the patient's
> head - to her left.
>
> Dr Fowler spoke to the patient briefly, telling her that he
> had brought some 'young doctors' to see her. When he had
> finished speaking, the physician nodded to Heather Muir as a
> sign for her to start speaking herself. Heather did so, and
> as she did, the patient turned her head to the left to look
> at her. Dr Fowler laughed, and apologised that this hadn't
> worked. He explained that he had not been expecting the
> patient to react to anything on her left.

The subsequent development of this teaching session went on to show that
the diagnosis implied by the consultant's little trick was
substantiated. But the point is that he had been able to plan the
performance in the first place on the basis of his prior knowledge of
the diagnosis - and hence of the likely outcome of the demonstration.
In this case the physician managed to pass off his failure - he was able

to laugh it off.

I noted that failures in stage management of this sort did tend to produce occasions for laughter between students and staff. Sometimes, it would be a source for covert mirth and sniggering from the students - a sort of *schadenfrevde* and a delight in their teachers' deflation and possible loss of composure. Alternatively - as in the example above - it could be a topic of humour shared between teacher and students.

In the following example the patient was an elderly man, whom we saw in an acute poisoning unit. The patient had taken an overdose of a drug prescribed to him to control hypertension - he had thus drastically reduced his blood pressure. Since coming into hospital he had also started showing symptoms of alcohol dependence. He had now recovered sufficiently to be sitting up in an armchair, but presented a sorry appearance, and gave a general impression of being confused and disoriented.

> The patient had a black eye, and when Dr Ewing asked him how he had got it, he went into a rambling account of how he had been set upon by the ward orderly so he could 'keep his job open' - there having been no other patients in the ward at that time....

> Dr Ewing asked him the date, the day of the week, and the year, and he got them all correct. The doctor then encouraged him to elaborate on his story of assault by the orderly. But the patient did not attempt to offer any more detail; or to embroider his story in any way.

> Dr Ewing said that some patients of this sort show 'micrographia' - that is their handwriting gets very small. He gave Mr W. a notebook and a ballpoint, and asked him to write his name and address. The patient did this very laboriously. But when we examined it, although there was clear evidence of tremor, there was no sign of the handwriting getting any smaller....

Later Dr Ewing took the students into a side room to talk about the patient:

> ...whilst talking about the symptoms of 'confabulation' (i.e. making up stories and fantasies), Dr Ewing said that he had been trying to get Mr W. to confabulate further about his imagined assault (he had in fact received his injury by falling out of bed during an episode of delerium tremens). Dr Ewing went on that he hadn't really been confabulating - and he would 'see him afterwards'; similarly, while talking about the patient's failure to display micrographia, he said he clearly hadn't 'briefed Mr W. properly beforehand!'

The physician and the students all laughed at this overt reference to the 'pre-diagnosed' nature of cold medicine bedside teaching. The context was a potentially disturbing one - an acute poisoning unit, where a number of parasuicides were being cared for. It was a depressing place - physically unprepossessing as well as occasioning emotional response for the patients. Tension and nervous laughter were never far beneath the surface. However, Dr Ewing's joke at this point came off in terms of his explicit reference to the 'stage management' of the encounter. His comment represented a glimpse behind the scenes, and a glimpse of the stage machinery whereby a performance of clinical technique could be sustained. In this instance, nature failed to mimic art and the physician's reliance on his foreknowledge of the patient's condition let him down.

Students acknowledge the physician's prior information about the patient as a resource in demonstrating his clinical skill and producing 'neat' diagnostic findings. I made the following notes after a coffee time discussion on Dr Burton's teaching style and personality. The fourth year students were sitting with two men in their Final Phase.

'The students had been commenting on Dr Burton's claim to be able to diagnose a myocardial infarction simply from his observation of cyanosis about the patient's features. A fair degree of incredulity was expressed as to whether Dr Burton really could produce accurate diagnoses, as he claimed.

A senior student said that the consultants often pretended to be making a diagnosis on the strength of what they were doing at the bedside with the juniors, but in fact had access to extra information which they didn't acknowledge. John (a fourth year) agreed, and said that when Dr Burton had examined a patient he'd never seen before he'd been completely stumped. He instanced the 18 year old girl we had seen with symptoms and signs of a neurological disorder'.

This patient had caused a certain amount of comment among the students. The consultant had taken a teaching session on a girl who had been admitted the previous evening. He had not actually studied her himself, and it appeared that no diagnosis had yet been formulated. Certainly the doctor had no previous diagnosis to rely on. We came upon the patient as a senior student was taking her history. Dr Burton got the senior to present the case to the clinique. The history was a fairly vague one of numbness, tingling and weakness of the limbs. Dr Burton asked the girl some questions himself and then went on to perform an examination of the patient. He concentrated on a neurological examination of her arms and legs.

When he had completed demonstrating the examination, Dr Burton commented that the clinical findings were hard to interpret and he had never seen a case like it before. The doctor commented to the senior student: would he like this case in his final examination? The student said he would not and the doctor agreed he would not either. As the students commented subsequently, faced with a totally fresh patient the consultant was in difficulties. He was unable to provide the display of diagnostic wizardry which was something of a trademark of his teaching style. (Subsequently the girl's trouble was tentatively identified as disseminated sclerosis, although when I enquired later this was still far from certain).

I am not implying that there was any incompetence on the doctor's part: I have no external criteria to discover whether the case really needed to be as puzzling as he made it. Rather I am pointing out how the circumstances of his teaching session made it a topic for student conversation. Whether or not they were justified in their implied criticism, it provided an apt illustration of their recognition of this feature of 'cold' medicine.

It is by virtue of the 'prediagnosis' of patients' conditions that clinicians may select patients for the demonstration of specific features of history taking, examinations and diagnosis. In many teaching sessions at the bedside, lengthy examinations are curtailed, and the teaching physician or surgeon will indicate at the outset of the direction in which students' enquiries should go. They may tell them to begin with that the patient has had a particular sort of presenting trouble and ask the students to question the patient on that basis - concentrating their questioning on that system rather than taking a complete history. They may even dispense with a history altogether and direct the students to go straight on to the physical examination of a particular system.

This sort of management of the teaching session is well illustrated in the pedagogical approach used in one clinique, known as the 'Friday run around'. Here students were given a list of patients whom they were to visit briefly, and examine just one thing about them, or ask them about just one aspect of their illness. Here is a typical set of instructions issued to the student members of the clinique before they left the teaching room to 'run around' the wards. The consultant put up a list of patients' names with the instructions beside them, and diagrams of the wards, giving the locations of the patients' beds in them:

Male, 1st Floor

(1)	J.	axial skeleton
(2)	B.	had pancreatitis - take history
(3)	Thos. R.	examine abdomen
(4)	Jas. R.	examine ocular movements

Female, 2nd Floor

| (1) | S. | examine precordium |
| (2) | D. | "   " |

A subsequent 'run around' offers a very similar picture:

Male

(1)	R.	examine precordium
(2)	L.	lesion by left groin
(3)	P.	alcoholic - take it from there

Female

(1)	H.	right eye
(2)	H.	Parkinsonism - find out about it
(3)	F.	examine abdomen
(4)	P.	examine left eye
(5)	C.	presented with haemoptysis - find out why

Having received their 'marching orders' in this way, the students split up and go about individually, visiting the various patients on their list. Subsequently they all come back to the teaching room and compare notes on what they discovered with some of the physicians.

These exercises provide students with excellent opportunities for

observing the particularities of specified conditions. They would
normally engage enthusiastically in the performance of these 'run
arounds'; they combined variety with the ability to gain diagnostic
information (or confirmation) with least effort. This variety of
diagnostic 'game' is, as I have said, made possible by virtue of the
clinicians' detailed knowledge of the patients which they have already
assembled in the course of their routine diagnostic and therapeutic
work. In such situations they can, to all intents and purposes,
guarantee that if the students enquire and observe methodically, then
clinical 'facts' are there for the finding.

   On the other hand, for the 'game' to be successful and a satisfying
one, then the information should not be entirely 'obvious', simply by
virtue of the preliminary information provided. As has already been
described, the process of educational 'cold' medicine can be spoiled if
the discovery of clinical information is short circuited. Such short
circuiting can arise also when patients are selected for spot diagnostic
exercises. If the exercise is too specific, then the 'answer' may turn
out to be a 'foregone conclusion'. This can be exemplified in the
following incident, taken from my field notes in medicine.

   One morning, I discovered that 'mock' final examinations were
   being conducted on the wards, and the junior students were
   rather at a loose end. This was explained to me by Owens,
   who commented to me that since they had not been allocated
   any patients to 'clerk' this week, they were having to 'fill
   in with lesser tasks'. This morning, he told me, they had
   been given 'little missions' to occupy them for the first
   hour or so. Owens told me that he had been told to go and
   see a woman patient and diagnose what was wrong with her just
   by listening to her voice. He told me, with an air of some
   disgust, that there was only one condition that can be
   diagnosed just from the voice. 'What is that?' I asked him.

   'Myxoedema'.

   'What's that?'

   'Thyroid deficiency'.

   'And what happens to the voice?' I asked him.

   'It gets low, and slow, and monotonous, and the syllables
   get mixed....' (he himself imitated the low monotone).
   '...if she hasn't got that I shall refuse to make a diagnosis.

   He left to visit 'his' patient.

   One by one the students on the unit came in and went off on
   their various 'missions', while I stayed in the teaching room,
   writing up my notes and chatting to students as they came and
   went. A bit later, Owens came back, and said in a bored, I
   told you so voice, 'She had a slow, monotonous voice....'

   In this instance it appeared that despite the ingenuity of suggesting
that the student should diagnose from the patient's voice alone, the
instruction was too 'obvious', gave away too much information in itself,
and - for the student concerned - undermined what he saw as the purpose
of the exercise.

These diagnostic exercises, with their game like characteristics introduce us to the theme of the next chapter. That is, the stage management of routine bedside teaching encounters.

6 Versions of Clinical Medicine

As I have already suggested, the overt rationale of the clinical phase of professional training is that the novice is thereby exposed to 'practice' in the context of 'real' work. This is certainly the way in which clinical training in medicine is thought of, and the students welcome their clinical work in that spirit. This chapter will explore some of the ways in which that 'reality' is managed, so that certain versions of medical work and medical knowledge are portrayed to the students.

HOT AND COLD MEDICINE

One morning I was standing with a small group of students who had been taking histories from patients, either individually or in pairs. As we hung about in the corridor we were joined by one of the female patients. She immediately began to complain about 'her' patient. As the student had started to take the history, the patient had immediately told her that she had mitral stenosis, as a complication of rheumatic fever contracted in childhood. She had, the student complained, 'spoiled all the fun'. This episode, and its connotations of a spoiled encounter, gave me an *entrée* into the problem of social order at the bedside. The feature which emerges in this context is the diagnosed nature of patients in the course of morning teaching rounds; their trouble has been at least differentially diagnosed, and the diagnosis may in fact be considered definitive by the hospital clinicians. Management of some sort will have been initiated, tests ordered, procedures undertaken. Symptoms such as severe pain will have been controlled if possible, and physical signs such as high fever or blood loss may have abated or disappeared altogether.

This aspect of the teaching round is recognised by students. They contrast it with cases that they see on waiting nights. In student jargon, the distinction is sometimes characterised as a difference between 'hot' and 'cold' medicine. One the one hand, 'hot' medicine is seen as exposing the students to 'real' medicine: histories are being taken for the first time and are crucial to the patient's treatment; the illness must be managed and diagnosis attempted. There is a sense of the dramatic, the unpredictable, and the rough and tumble of acute hospital medicine. 'Cold' medicine, on the other hand, is seen and characterised as 'contrived', and carefully managed encounters; they lack the same sense of immediacy and unpredictability.

The bedside teaching session ('cold medicine') is a social encounter which is constructed in such a way as to simulate a supposed 'reality' of normal medical work ('hot medicine'). I have indicated some ways in which the situation is located in a medical context - and thus resembles the 'real world'; I shall go on to discuss how it differs.

Although a history may have been elicited from the patient on a number of previous occasions, in the course of 'cold', bedside teaching, the students may be asked to take one yet again.

e.g., The patient said at one point, 'Half the students here have
      seen me before, and my history is as big as that....' He
      held his hands apart to indicate a thick pile of notes.

and

      The patient interjected that she had told her story so
      often that 'I should have brought along a tape recording'.

This distinction is remarked by students in their perceptions of
their waiting nights. As one student expressed it to me:

      I went to three and watched what they were doing. You were
      there while the actual history was being taken, not
      listening to it for the tenth time.

And another girl offered the following recommendation of waiting nights
as educational experiences: 'Seeing things as they happen rather than
being taught on things once everything's been decided'.

Attendance on waiting nights allows the students to become more
involved, at first hand, in the therapeutic work of the ward personnel.
They are, so to speak, 'in on the act'. As one girl put it, 'It was
good on waiting nights - they included us'. Students see things as they
are done, and can see for themselves the practical significance of
clinical procedures.

The students thus get a chance to participate more directly in the
clinical staff's work with the patients who arrive in the wards. Even
when staff members are too busy to stop and 'teach' on the new
patients, the students whose turn it is to spend the evening with them
can still be present; they can look over the shoulder of junior doctors
or senior students as they admit patients and perform the initial
clinical tasks of diagnosis and management. In contrast with the work
of clinical teaching in the mornings, the students also get some
opportunity to do things for themselves, as well as seeing things done.
They can 'have a go' at such simple procedures as drawing off a blood
sample.

Since what happens on waiting nights depends upon the unforeseen and
unforeseeable intake of new patients, what the students can actually
see and do on any particular night is variable and unpredictable. On
the mornings after waiting nights it is a normal topic of conversation
for the rest of the members of the clinique to ask those who had been in
for an account of what had happened. Often they have to report that
little or nothing occurred. Sometimes only one patient was admitted
during the hours that students spent on the wards. They can find
themselves 'hanging about' with no dramatic events to engage their
interest. For instance, I was chatting with a group of students at the
end of the morning's teaching:

      I asked Brian if they had been into theatre very much and
      he said that they had, especially on waiting nights, when
      one of them would scrub up and assist at the operation.
      Margaret added that waiting nights were the only time when
      they learned anything. Harriet interrupted him, saying
      that that depended on there being anything happening. One
      of the other girls said, 'Oh, didn't you have anything?'

Harriet admitted that when she had been in, there had been no new admissions, and so little or nothing for the students to do with themselves. In an interview one of the male students offered the following account of his first experience of coming in on a waiting night:

'The first waiting night was appalling. It says on the noticeboard that you're expected to attend waiting night from seven to nine. I arrived at seven and nothing was happening. Admittedly not many patients had been admitted...so we went down to A and E [Accident and Emergency] on our own, and saw the one patient that had been admitted. Then we went to the pub...we came back later, but only cuts and bruises had come in'.

Although he was complaining partly about the organisational arrangements of the unit he was on, the lack of admissions clearly also limited what the students could see and do even on their own initiative. On the other hand, students may find themselves with plenty to do as patients come in during the evening. This is reflected in the following report from a student who was attached to a surgical unit at the time:

Sean talked to me about waiting nights. With nine members of the clinique, and a term of ten weeks, since the students came to waiting night three at a time, it meant that they were only supposed to attend three waiting nights altogether. Sean told me that last time he had stayed from three o'clock in the afternoon until three o'clock the following morning: there had been things happening all that time. He hadn't noticed the time pass, as there had been so much to occupy him - going backwards and forwards between the operating theatre and the Accident and Emergency department. He had been asked if he would like to admit a patient, and he gave a pantomime of the enthusiasm with which he had accepted the offer of the chance to do so.

On occasion students find themselves pitched into the most dramatic and critical sort of medical incident. One student was on the wards one evening when there were two cardiac arrests simultaneously; he found himself thumping a patient's chest in an attempt to resuscitate him. (Although he managed to break some ribs in the course of the external cardiac massage, he was unable to save the patient).

The 'hot' medicine which students see on their waiting night visits may be rather different from what they are used to from the normal morning teaching rounds. As I have already indicated, although patients may still be very sick indeed, by the time they are on the wards, their most alarming and distressing symptoms will generally have been controlled to some extent. By and large, the ward at ten o'clock in the morning presents an orderly appearance. Although the ward may be extremely busy, the patients themselves are mostly in a quiet and stable state. Either tucked up under the bedclothes, sitting in their armchairs or pottering about between the rows of beds, the patients do not normally present a picture of distress and disorder.

The waiting nights are of especial relevance to students attached to

surgical units. For surgical cliniques, waiting nights provide prime
opportunities for students to go into the operating theatres and observe
emergency operations as they are done.   In this way, students see
things that are rather different from what they see on the wards, and
they can act as informal channels of clinical information for the other
students. Not only can students observe surgery on such occasions; they
may also be allowed to come onto the theatre floor and scrub up, and
assist at an operation. Thus one girl proudly described to me how on
one waiting night she had held a retractor for two and a half hours: she
had been assisting at an operation on a middle-aged man for a vagotomy
and pyloroplasty. She described how she had watched five operations
being carried out, and had 'enjoyed it thoroughly'.

Students' perspectives on the immediacy and 'freshness' of the
medicine and surgery they see on waiting nights can be contrasted with
the managed nature of the patients' conditions that they see on the
majority of other teaching occasions. One boy contrasted the two
contexts in describing his experiences in surgery; we were chatting
together on the coach on the way out to one of the 'peripheral'
hospitals:

> 'After waiting nights', he said, 'Mr Michael takes the
> students to see the new admissions. If you've already seen
> the patient, you keep quiet while Mr Michael plays games
> with the others, and sees how well they can make a diagnosis.
> Then you fill in the details - and try desperately to
> remember which abdomen it was, when you've only seen a
> little bit of it in theatre'.

This student thus drew attention to the contrivance of bedside
teaching periods, and the reality of what happened at waiting nights,
when the diagnosis was first formulated. He describes the nature of
the 'morning after' teaching as 'playing games' and 'false'. One of
the female students on a medical attachment made a very similar point
to me in the course of an interview:

> In fact by the time we get round to clerking them it's
> really rather ridiculous because, mostly, they've been
> treated and all their symptoms - all their signs certainly,
> and some of the symptoms - have gone. And it's also about
> the eighth time they've told their story and they're
> beginning to abbreviate it a bit by the time they get
> round to you....In fact I get a lot more out of going to
> waiting nights and clerking patients with one of the final
> phase students. That's when you get a bit of the
> excitement of diagnosis - nobody really knows.

NON THERAPEUTIC ENCOUNTERS

The bedside teaching encounter differs from 'normal' medical
interactions in that it is not therapeutic.   Specifically designed for
teaching purposes, this session is not part of the patient's treatment.
Bedside teaching is sometimes spoken of as having a beneficial function
for some patients - in terms of keeping them occupied and relieving the
boredom of long hours in bed. In that sense it can be therapeutic -
but not in terms of the usual processes of diagnosis and management of
clinical medicine and surgery. It is occasionally stated by clinicians

that there is always the possibility that new information about the
patient can be thrown up in the course of bedside teaching and
clerking. This does occasionally happen. In discussing with me what
had given him the greatest personal satisfaction over the year, one
student told me:

> 'In the second term of medicine, I did take a history from
> somebody and I found that they had been taking an overdose
> of some tablets...and I didn't think other people had got
> that from their history; and the guy said, "Would you do
> further investigation - because you found that: look at
> her urine or anything like that?" I found she had...
> (inaudible)...nephritis, I think it was. And that was
> through that, so that was rewarding I suppose in a way'.

This was the only example I found of a student's work, either in
clerking, or during bedside teaching sessions, where his or her
enquiries appeared to provide important new information on the patient's
condition. On a few other occasions students provided additional
information but it did not give important new insights into the
diagnosis or management - rather they produced confirmatory evidence for
decisions already taken.

> Sometimes they'll tell you things behind the doctor's back
> - they'll tell you things that they haven't told the
> doctors. One time at the (peripheral) Hospital a lady was
> telling me about her drinking habits. I don't know if
> she'd told the doctors or not - but she told me that she
> was telling me on the side because she didn't want the
> doctors to know. She drank about three or four bottles of
> sherry a day.
>
> P.A. Did you tell the doctors?
>
> Yes. I think they knew she was more or less an alcoholic,
> but not how much she drank.

Similarly, a student spotted something new during a medical teaching
round. We were at the bedside of an old man: the session was conducted
primarily as a history taking exercise. But one of the students - no
doubt using the powers of observation, as he had been taught - looked at
the patient's hands, and thought he noticed 'finger clubbing'. He asked
the physician about this, and she examined the patient's hand for
herself. She agreed that there did indeed appear to be some clubbing
present, and drew the attention of the rest of the group to it. She
added that she had not previously noticed that herself. She
complimented the student on his observation, but it was clear that this
new sign was not important, and in no way modified the diagnosis.

It is an even rarer occurrence for a student to suggest a form of
therapy that has not been considered by the clinicians, and have the
suggestion acted upon. I came across only one isolated incident of this
nature. I missed the actual occurrence, but I was on the ward the day
after. When I arrived the students were standing about, waiting for a
surgeon to come and teach them. They were teasing one of their number
(Keith Foster). When I asked what the fuss was about they explained
that during an out patient session, the consultant had not been sure of
the best treatment for a woman patient and Keith Foster had made a
suggestion which the surgeon had accepted. This had been noted by the
students as a 'star' performance. As he himself explained to me

afterwards:

> My mother, she's approaching menopause just now and she'
> having terrible menorrhagia...and flushing - her face al
> flushing when she least wants it to - and so her doctor
> put her on phenobarbitone because it reduces the oestroge
> to acceptable levels....When thin g s like that are sort of
> personal to me I tend to think it over...and whenever the
> question arose of how to cut down the level of circulatin
> oestrogens in this woman, I just thought of phenobarbitone.
> I didn't tell anyone else that - I wanted to look smart.

Because of this student's personal experience, he did appear 'smart'
to the consultant surgeon and to his fellow students. The fact that it
became such a topic of conversation and teasing among the members of the
clinique indicates just how rare and noteworthy such an event was -
indeed, almost unheard of.

PUTTING THE CLOCK BACK

In discussing the nature of 'cold' medicine at the bedside I emphasised
how it can be contrasted with the 'hot' situation that students
encountered on waiting nights. At this point I shall develop the
argument in terms of the passage of time in relation to students'
contact with the patients on the wards - and again, consider some ways
in which the maintenance of the situation may be problematic for the
members concerned. When 'cold' medicine is encountered, the patient's
hospital career is already under way, and his or her diagnostic identity
may be firmly fixed. Yet for the purposes of the teaching exercise the
passage of time must be discounted. There may be an attempt to 'put the
clock back' and treat the patient as if there had been no intervening
period and thus threaten the reality of the diagnostic exercise by
divulging this information.

In addition to the patients' and doctors' information state concerning
the illness - the shared knowledge about the patient - there is also
the fact that the nature of the patient's illness will change over
time. Thus, it becomes a problem of cold medicine that, with the
passage of time, the initial signs and symptoms of the presenting
complaint diminish or disappear.

Patients who are admitted to the wards on waiting nights with, for
example, myocardiac infarction or respiratory failure in medicine, or
acute abdominal pain or urine retention in surgery, regularly display
accentuated clinical signs and symptoms. The myocardiac infarction
will be in pain, short of breath, cyanosed and so on. The patient with
acute abdominal pain may be vomiting, display a distended abdominal
region and so on. On waiting nights, the students attending the ward
will see the patients' distress and the clear indications of their
conditions. Yet by the time the bulk of regular ward teaching takes
place, things have changed. The use of analgesics, for instance, will
mean that severe pain will routinely be diminished. Similarly the
acute signs and symptoms of respiratory failure, high fever, or blood
loss will have been remedied by appropriate treatment soon after
admission.

We passed on to another woman who was lying curled up in bed
with a cage over her legs. Dr Burton took his stethoscope
and listened at the apex of her chest, and then got the
students to do so. He commented to Jane Peters - who had
been in on the previous night - that the breath sounds had
changed considerably since the woman's admission on the
previous day, and she agreed that there were certain
differences. Dr Burton pointed out that the patient had
been on penicillin for just twelve hours, but that it was
already taking effect.

Or again, during the same morning's teaching we spent some time at the
bedside of an elderly male patient.

The patient (who was himself a retired GP) recognised two of
the members of the round as the housemen who had admitted
him the previous night. One of them described to us that
this patient's neck veins had been 'sticking out like tree
trunks'. We all looked at the neck veins, but they did not
appear to be distended at all.

The abatement of signs presents problems for the clinical teacher.
When he comes to demonstrate a point of diagnostic observation, the
signs which he wishes to show the students may well elude him
altogether.

Dr Miller reminded us that anaemic patients often have a dry,
red, swollen tongue. He asked Miss M. to put out her tongue:
it looked quite normal. 'I'm very disappointed', the doctor
said, 'On Saturday she had a red, swollen tongue'.

Such contingencies may spoil the clinician's smooth production of a
teaching display. Thus on one occasion, a consultant was attempting
to display the elicitation of nystagmus - involuntary flickering
movement of the eyes. Although the consultant appeared satisfied that
there was some nystagmus present it was by no means marked. In the
middle of teaching on this first patient, he therefore charged off,
taking the students and me with him, and took us off to another ward
and a new patient. He immediately started to test the new patient's
eyes, and was clearly crestfallen when this patient no longer displayed
the nystagmus he had expected to see. Anticlimax was total. The
reason for the disappearance of nystagmus in this case was not clear;
signs and symptoms can abate spontaneously, and not as any obvious
consequence of the therapy that patients have received.

e.g.After a lengthy discussion of polycythaemia - based partly
on a run-through of a report of a blood film taken from the
patient, and ending with comments on possible treatment,
Dr Cowan concluded, 'Unfortunately, Mr G's next two blood
counts are bloody normal'. 'Without treatment?' one or two
of the students asked. Dr Cowan confirmed, 'Without
treatment'.

Such a contingency is doubly problematic for clinical teaching. In the
first place, the spontaneous remission of a sign impedes the diagnostic
'game'; but secondly, it does not even provide occasion for a
demonstration and affirmation of the efficacy of approved therapy. At
least in my earlier example, the consultant could sidetrack from
diagnostic signs to the swift and beneficial action of penicillin. In

the present context, even that alternative is not open.

These aspects of the accomplishment of clinical teaching clearly illustrate the divergent relevancies of therapeutic and educational work in the hospital. On the one hand, there is the physician's concern for treating the patient - effecting a cure, or at least palliation of his symptoms. On the other hand, the physician also has concerns relevant to his teaching, where his routine clinical work may be in conflict with his immediate educational objectives. Thus the doctor's 'disappointment' over the patient's tongue, or the 'unfortunately' in the episode above can be seen as oriented to the relevance for clinical teaching. The abatement of diagnostic signs therefore presents a crucial problem in the successful production of a clinical 'mock up'. It is hard to sustain the bedside teaching session as an approximately to 'real' diagnostic work when the physical manifestations that would determine such diagnosis are missing or masked. Therapeutic success can spell educational difficulty.

The development of the patient's career and the episodic interruptions of bedside teaching periods becomes a particularly crucial feature in the teaching of surgery, and students' perceptions of that subject. In some ways, the distinction between 'hot' and 'cold' medicine becomes acute in this context. For students, the vivid drama of acute work is highlighted in the surgical admission, and the immediate involvement in the operating theatre. Waiting nights provide the main chance of students' presence at such 'hot' situations. Yet it is often the case that after this 'dramatic' intervention, matters go very cold indeed. For, after the operation, there may be little or nothing of the original lump or lesion for the students to see. Once it has been cut out or repaired, there is only a fresh wound to observe, and the paraphernalia of post operative care, such as drips, drains and so on. It was an important part of students' perceptions of surgery, as against medicine, that apart from waiting nights, there was little or nothing for them to see, and thus reduced scope for undertaking diagnosis.

There is a distinction to be drawn between the trajectories of the patient career as between medical and surgical cases. Whereas in both situations the patient passes from 'hot' to 'cold', the shape of such a passage differs. For most medical cases, signs, symptoms and so on diminish by degrees; even after intensive care, patients may be on displaying signs. For most surgical cases, the intervention of such surgery marks a sharp break in the illness trajectory. The course of the trouble is routinely charted in terms of pre and post operative phases, and reckoned in post operative days. There is, in general, no sharp division in the medical patient's hospital career. (Here I am of course concerned only with the 'in-patient' phase of the overall patient career. For cases of both types, the admission to the hospital ward marks a sharply defined status passage).

An alternative way of expressing this is to point out that the students' contact with patients is typically episodic and intermittent. The bedside teaching session represents one interlude in the course of the patient's career, as it is negotiated over time. (Indeed, it is often seen as 'time out' for the patients - as a possibly entertaining session and a relief from the boredom of life on the ward).

Some patients are visited only once during their stay in hospital.

One of the tasks to be done in a teaching period is to produce an account of the patient's career and the trajectory of his illness. As we have seen, there may be an attempt to discount the passage of time and to reconstitute it from the beginning - by taking a history if the patient were being newly admitted. Yet, in addition, the relevant information may no longer be retrievable in that manner.

In the light of the problem of the abatement of signs, a further theme can be introduced. This concerns the way in which the clinician teaches by means of a retrospective appeal to his own knowledge of the patient's prior condition. This arises from two contingencies of the passage of time. Firstly, the clinician may encounter the problem of the abatement of diagnostic clues, as I have already outlined. Alternatively, it may happen that, with repetition, the patient's telling of his own story changes. The doctor will have an understanding of the patient's illness, based on previous clinical work, and histories elicited on previous occasions. Problems are therefore created if the patient's history - part of the evidence for the doctor's formulation of the illness - now appears to be at odds with that which originally informed the diagnosis. On the one hand, changes in the patient's history may simply be a reflection of forgetfulness, as some items are now felt with less immediate impact by the sick person. They may simply 'cut corners' in presenting their history repeatedly - and, in 'tidying it up' and getting it 'off pat', they may unwittingly omit information: information which they hear as irrelevant detail, but which the doctor and students might hear as important diagnostic indications.

Alternatively, the patient may attempt to 'improve' upon his original history - and add or subtract information in accordance with what the doctor is thought to be seeking. As Turner points out:

> Conceivably...the 'repetition' of the therapist's request for an account may be taken by patients as a rejection of accounts given to date, and as signifying that the patient has yet to adequately answer the question, 'Why are you here?' (Turner, 1972).

If the patient, then, in the face of repeated requests for his story, should hear these requests in such a way, then he may come to doctor his own history in a search for one which will pass muster as an adequate account. The history is repeated in terms of 'Will this do?', and in the telling of it, it is changed from occasion to occasion.

Additionally, we must also note the possibility of forms of 'deviance disavowal' as patients rewrite their medical biography. Again, as severely disabling or distressing symptoms are less in evidence, patients may come to 'normalise' their condition in retrospect. They may make light of matters such as pain, which previously they made much of, as they underplay the severity of their own problem. Such normalisation may be a stratagem designed to alleviate patients' own anxieties, or to express the desire not to be 'too much trouble' to the hospital staff (cf. Davis, 1961, 1963).

For a number of reasons, then, the complaint as it now appears or as it is now described, may differ significantly from the original presentation. It is in the face of such occurrences that the teaching doctor can invoke the 'in fact' clause. Discrepancies are rectified, and the possibly competing accounts - of the doctor and his patient -

are shown to be an artefact of the lapse of time rather than a failure of diagnostic procedure. An instance of this occurred during a history taking exercise with a senior house officer and an elderly male patient. The old man was very hard of hearing, and was described by the houseman as being 'not the best of historians'. I noted after this session:

> (In response to questioning from one of the students) the
> patient reported that he had not been having to pass water
> many times during the day. But Dr May commented, 'In fact,
> he reported frequency during the day as well....' She also
> explained that he had been sick the day before he came in,
> although on admission he did not report vomiting.

In this instance, then, the doctor repairs the discrepancy by reference to the patient's general failing as a historian - exemplified by a further retrospective appeal to his inaccuracy concerning his nausea when he was admitted to the hospital.

The clinicians' use of appeals to what was 'in fact' the case also draws attention to a further consideration with regard to time. As time passes and the patient's hospital career develops, then - in the great majority of cases - the hospital personnel will become more certain of their diagnosis and the appropriate therapy. Tests, procedures and observation, coupled with the results of any treatment that may have been initiated, will normally rule out at least some of the possibilities entertained under an initial differential diagnosis; more specific lines of reasoning will be confirmed.

The distinction between uncertainty and certainty over diagnoses is an important dimension in the evaluation of the 'hot' medicine of waiting nights and 'cold' bedside teaching sessions. When patients are admitted in the acute phase of their illness, the clinicians may not be in a position to state a definitive diagnosis. As time goes on, and the patient's hospital career progresses, the chances are that the diagnosis will tend to become more certain, (it is not necessarily so; some conditions will go on puzzling the doctors and a definitive diagnosis may never be reached). From the students' viewpoint, we have already seen how 'hot' situations may provide occasions for a greater degree of involvement in clinical work on their part. Additionally, when we consider the pedagogical aspects, it follows that the discourse of hot medicine may be marked by a greater degree of negotiation between the student(s) and the teacher. The interaction may take a form which approaches more closely a 'team effort' in arriving at differential diagnoses. These often have to be couched in terms of 'wait and see'; further decision making has to wait upon the outcome of tests and procedures, the efficacy of therapy, or further questioning of the patient. The patient's condition may be clear, in general terms (e.g., respiratory failure) but detailed investigation of the sociology and seriousness of the condition may have to be postponed until after the management of the initial crisis. In any event, the clinician will be unlikely to possess as full a knowledge of the 'right' answers as he will when the patient is seen in the course of a normal morning teaching round. In general, then, the development of the patient's career will be marked by a move from relative negotiability towards relative certainty. The social relationships implied by this distribution of knowledge will, correspondingly, shift from a relatively egalitarian one to one in which the distance between the teacher and the taught is emphasised. This process can be illustrated in the following field notes taken from my observations in surgery. The first extract was noted on the day the patient in question was admitted; the second was made on the day after his admission, by which time the patient has been operated on. On the first day, there was agreement in <u>general</u> as to patient's condition, but some uncertainty as to its precise nature. After surgery the position, as far as the surgeons were concerned, was much clearer.

Day one

Mr Jackson took us into the ward, telling us he was taking us to see someone who had come in during the day. The patient was an elderly man (73), and he looked pretty ill as he lay in bed.

We all gathered round the bedside the Mr Jackson spoke to the patient. He asked him what had made him come in to the hospital. He replied (with some difficulty) that he had pain, indicating his abdomen. Mr Jackson asked if he had had any trouble with his stomach previously; he said that he had had 'a lot of gas' over the previous year, and had hiccoughed a lot. The surgeon asked him if he had been taking any pills or powders for his stomach. The patient said he hadn't. Mr Jackson asked him if he was in pain now, and the patient told us that he was. (Certainly he appeared to be in considerable discomfort, wincing and grimacing as he talked).

Mr Jackson then took back the bedclothes. He pointed to an old scar low on the patient's abdomen. 'Was that for a prostrate?'. The patient confirmed that it was. Mr Jackson then palpated the abdomen; the patient said it was sore and painful all over.

Mr Jackson told the patient 'It's beginning to look as if you're going to have to have an operation'. He put back the bedclothes, and shepherded us off into the doctors' room, where there were three X-ray films displayed. As we stood around, Dr Richards - who was already in the room - spoke to Mr Jackson and they discussed the timing of the operations that they were going to be doing. Mr Jackson then turned to the films and asked the students what they could see. Several of them simultaneously pointed out that there appeared to be air under the right side of the diaphragm. Mr Jackson asked what that meant. Somebody volunteered, 'A burst duodenal ulcer', while Redmond muttered 'Ruptured viscus'. Mr Jackson asked him to repeat what he had said; he said he'd just said 'a ruptured viscus'. Mr Jackson agreed that it could be any ruptured organ, not necessarily the duodenum. Alan Cartwright suggested that it might be the bladder - considering that he'd had the prostactectomy; it might have become blocked again and burst. Mr Jackson pointed out that the bladder is outside the peritoneum, and doesn't contain air anyway. Mr Jackson asked what else it could be. Somebody volunteered that it might be a diverticulum. Mr Jackson agreed, and said that he would put his money on this patient having a ruptured diverticulum.

Redmond asked about the patient's pain in his left shoulder. Mr Jackson appeared to misinterpret the question - saying that

it was just derived from the irritated diaphragm. Redmond
said, Yes, he understood that, but queried the pain in the
left shoulder when the air appeared to be under the right
side. Mr Jackson pointed to the X-ray, saying that it
couldn't really be seen, but he thought that there would
probably be air on the left hand side as well. He commented
that he had asked the patient about the pain in his shoulder
'with the prior knowledge' of having seen the X-ray pictures.

Before discussing this episode, let us go straight on to the notes I
took on the following day:

Day two

[In the course of a teaching round] we went to see the
patient we had seen yesterday with Mr Jackson. Mr McBain
asked if anyone had seen this patient yesterday: of course
all of them had, and some of them mumbled that they had seen
him. Mr McBain picked on Anne Ogilvy to tell us what she
knew about the patient. She got all flustered and was
unable to present a coherent story. Mr McBain asked rather
sharply if Anne had examined the patient's abdomen, and
Redmond came to her rescue by pointing out that they had
only seen the patient for a few minutes the previous day.
....

We then went to the side room, where Mr McBain produced X-ray
film from the folder he had been carrying on the ward round.

He began by asking the students what they did when they came
in on waiting nights: did they just go round at seven
o'clock and then leave, or did they examine patients? He was
very critical in his manner and appeared to be commenting
specifically on the fact that none of them had examined the
patient on the previous day. The students defended themselves.
They pointed out that they did talk to patients and did
examine them, but pointed out that they had only seen him
briefly during the day, and in the evening he had been post-
operative.

Mr McBain then asked for comments on the X-ray pictures.
Redomond - repeating his comment of yesterday - said that the
air under the diaphragm suggested a ruptured viscus. 'Which
viscus?' the consultant asked. 'Any viscus'. Mr McBain was
not satisfied with this reply and wanted Redmond to commit
himself further.

There followed a rather confused discussion. Mr McBain could
see no reason for not believing the air to come from a
ruptured peptic ulcer. The students tried to persuade him
that Mr Jackson had told them that a diverticulum was more
probable, on the basis of the patient's age, and the sudden
onset of the trouble.

Mr McBain told them that it had been discovered since the
operation that the patient did have a history of ulceration
going back some twenty years - he had had barium meals and
so on. He also said that there would not be air released
from a diverticulum. Anne Ogilvy asked why this was. He
explained that it would be unlikely for a diverticulum to

'pop' - it was more likely for it to open gradually and form an abscess, which might then burst.

Mr McBain appeared to be totally unconvinced by the students' (admittedly incoherent) account of Mr Jackson's opinions of the previous day.

When I talked about what had happened subsequently, it appeared that some of the students began to have doubts about what had been said by the teaching surgeon on the first day. They too began to rewrite the patient's history, and bring the discussion into line with subsequent findings in the operating theatre.

This confusion, and the retrospective 'tidying up' of the accounts, highlights the way in which patients' histories and diagnoses can undergo transformation as their hospital career progresses. What is at issue here is not simply that surgery confirms or disconfirms differential diagnoses. What I wish to emphasise is the changing nature of the discourse and the students' position. The surgeon in the first extract used the language of betting, with the emphasis on the probabilities. On the second day, the surgeon was searching for greater certainty in the students' opinions. It must be emphasised that the students themselves were not privy to more information, although the surgeon himself was; nevertheless, their tentativeness was criticised by the surgeon from the vantage point of his own certainty. This is illustrated from the two clinicians' treatment of the suggestions offered. On day one, Mr Jackson led the discussion from the specific to the general, as he picked up on Redmond's suggestion of a 'ruptured viscus'. On day two, the same suggestion was treated very differently; now the surgeon insisted that students should commit themselves by plumping for specific diagnoses. Whereas, the first teaching session came off as a more collaborative venture, based upon a more egalitarian negotiation of the diagnosis, in the second, the surgeon tended to be much more dismissive of students' suggestions, which did not correspond to 'the facts of the case' as he knew them.

This last example provides us with some insight into the way in which clinical 'facts' are presented to students in the course of bedside teaching. This forms the theme of the next chapter, which explores some features of the social organisation of diagnosis and the perception of 'signs' and 'symptoms'.

7 Reproducing Illness

PERCEIVING ILLNESS

In the course of their diagnostic work, students find themselves working in a complex field of semiology - a field of manifestations which must be interpreted in order to produce a competent diagnostic picture, and to allow for the credible and warranted attribution of some label - that of a known disease or abnormality.

The conventional rhetoric of clinical medicine postulates two sorts of data available to the clinician at the bedside. They are referred to as 'signs' and 'symptoms'. Commonsensically the distinction between 'signs' and 'symptoms' is spoken of in terms of the distinction between 'objective' and 'subjective'. This distinction is employed by doctors, and indeed by sociological observers of medical practice. In Coe (1970, p.92), for instance, we find a contrast drawn between the disease and the patient's evaluation of his or her condition, between the signs, which 'may be objectively observed and even measurable, such as elevated body temperature or skin rash', and 'subjective symptoms such as a pain in the back'.

Although it is generally recognised that this may not be a hard and fast distinction, it is one which is generally employed in the occupational culture. The distinction corresponds roughly to the two clinical processes of 'taking a history' and 'performing an examination'. When the patient tells his or her story, and the doctor poses questions about the presenting complaint, then what is related will constitute the symptoms of the underlying disease. When the doctor turns to an examination of the patient's body - through observation, palpation, auscultation and so on - what is observed (seen, felt, heard, smelt) will be the signs of the disease. Further signs may be forthcoming if additional methods are used (X-rays, endoscopy, etc.), or if less direct inquiries are pursued (tests on the blood, urine, etc., sputum cultures and so on).

By and large sociologists of medicine have reflected this view in their work on so-called 'illness behaviour' - that is, in Mechanic's oft quoted formulation,

> On the most simple and obvious level, it is plain that symptoms are differentially perceived, evaluated, and acted upon (or not acted upon) by different kinds of people and in different social situations. (Mechanic, 1968, p.116)

The literature on illness behaviour is extensive (though its quality is not uniformly high). There is a common interest, however, in the examination of the actors' interpretation of their perceived biological changes and states. In other words, there is considerable emphasis on the 'subjective' aspect of 'illness', as opposed to what is assumed to be an objectively observable underlying 'disease'.

What tends to be lacking in the literature is a complementary concern
for the so called objective signs of disorders. Of course, our
language traps and beguiles us. Whereas our talk of subjectives states
immediately invites some consideration of sociological analysis of
interpretive procedures, talk of 'objective signs' seems to foreclose
any discussion of culturally influenced interpretation, of actors' own
understandings and so on. Insofar as such phenomena are regarded as
objective 'facts', then they tend to be taken on trust, and implicitly
exempted from sociological scrutiny.

Yet it is clear that what we see clearly now was not seen clearly at
other times (or not seen at all). What is patently obvious to members
of one culture may remain invisible to members of another. The
historical dimension to such 'seeing' is vividly illustrated by
Foucault (1963). His account of the birth of the clinic begins by
contrasting two descriptions of clinical observation, the first recorded
in the middle of the eighteenth century, the second less than a hundred
years later. The first describes in considerable detail the treatment
(successful, it was claimed) of a hysteric patient, who was forced to
bathe for hours each day for almost a year. At the end of the treatment
the clinician described the 'peeling away' of membranes, like 'damp
parchment', from various organs of the body. Foucault contrasts this
account with a nineteenth century description of a brain lesion, and the
'false membranes' frequently associated with chronic meningitis. The
detail of the description is closely analogous to that of the former
account. But as Foucault points out, the second description strikes us
as a careful, literal representation of a closely observed anatomical
phenomenon. The first strikes us today as downright bizarre, and the
phenomena which are listed do not tally with any observable physical
state recognised in contemporary anatomy and physiology. But both
report direct 'observations', of supposedly objective states of affairs.
Foucault uses the contrast between the two clinical descriptions to
illustrate the fundamental change which he associates with 'the birth of
the clinic'. In his terms, the change is dependent upon a change in the
nature of perception, which 'meant that the relation between the visible
and the invisible...changed its structure, revealing through gaze and
language what had previously been below their domain', while what was
previously treated as 'visible' became non events.

No doubt Foucault makes too much of the overall differences in
perception between different epochs. Many classic descriptions of
illnesses were produced well before the early nineteenth century, and
the 'birth of the clinic' did not mark a total 'paradigm shift' in all
areas of clinical observation and description. Nonetheless the
examples he selects do illustrate the fact that the apparently
'objective' observation of physical manifestations is itself socially
organised, culturally and historically bound.

Despite the claim that the clinical 'gaze' reveals openly and
directly, students find themselves having to learn how to perceive
competently. Throughout my time of observing clinical teaching there
were repeated occasions when there was considerable difficulty in the
recognition and reporting of clinical 'signs'. This applied to
perception with all the senses - and not merely the purely visual gaze.

This sort of problem was dramatically reflected in the following
incident. In the course of bedside teaching, the consultant told the

students that he wanted them all to listen to the patient's chest and
then come away from the bedside, one by one, and tell him what they had
found. While they were waiting to listen to the heart sounds and to
report their findings they were to draw diagrams of the 'classic'
auscultatory findings for a number of different conditions - mitral
stenosis, aortic stenosis and so on. The doctor then left the students
(and me) by the patient's bed and waited at the end of the ward for the
students to go to him and report their findings. As the doctor left,
Adrian Gray commented to us that, luckily for him, he had been working
at such things the night before, and so he was prepared for the task.
Adrian was the first to listen to the patient's chest, and having done
so he went off to report to the consultant. I stayed with the rest of
the group. When Adrian came back he spoke to John Finch, who asked him
what he had found. But Adrian said he was 'sworn to secrecy', although
he did let him copy down his recently revised 'classic findings'. He
did vouchsafe, however, that he had been given 'a bollocking' by the
consultant. One by one the students completed their brief examinations,
bending silently over him, and listening intently through their
stethescope (the patient himself said and did nothing). One by one they
left - reluctantly it appeared - and went to explain their findings to
the consultant. One by one they came back to the group by the patient's
bed, mostly with rather shamefaced expressions.   As they did so, and
began to compare notes, it became clear that whatever the 'classic'
manifestations, the students' hearing was by no means consistent with
what their teacher had expected. John Finch whispered to us that he had
been called 'a moron'; David Dean reported that he had been labelled 'a
buffoon'. They seemed to be rather amused by the dressing down that
they had all received. It emerged that a couple of them had correctly
identified some of the patient's distinctive signs, none of them had
produced a correct description of the overall pattern of heart sounds.
When they had all finished, the consultant physician returned, and had
them all have another listen to the patient's chest, to try to hear what
they had been supposed to hear in the first place.

Similar difficulty in perceiving can be illustrated in the following
extracts from my field notes:

> The students had been left to examine the patient's pulse,
> while Dr Richards went off for a moment or two to talk to
> Dr Goode. When Dr Richards came back to the members of
> the clinique he asked them to report the findings they had
> discovered.

> When the students were reporting their findings concerning
> the patient's pulse, there was some disagreement between
> them as to exactly what they had felt. In particular there
> was some disagreement as to whether what they had heard was
> in the following pattern:

> that is, whether there was a missed beat, or whether it was
> rather an ectopic beat followed by a compensatory gap:

> Similarly, when it came to a discussion of the patient's
> chest examination, there was even more disagreement. There

was no consensus as to whether there was presence or absence
of 'dullness' or percussion. Dr Richards 'took a vote on it',
percussed on his own account and used his 'chairman's casting
vote'.

One of the students in fact remarked to Dr Richards on this lack of
consensus - asking if they would in time all produce uniform
descriptions. Interestingly, Dr Richards interpreted his question as
referring to what was the best technique to use, rather than a problem
of the 'objectivity' of their findings.

Even in the apparently more straightforward context of visual
observation, things are not absolutely simple. Students often find it
hard adequately to formulate descriptions of 'appearances'. One of the
signs which students are continually called upon to 'notice' is the
complexion of the patient: the colour of a patient's skin is often
treated as a very useful diagnostic manifestation. But even in such
apparently mundane tasks as the description of a complexion, students
encounter difficulties. The following incident was by no means
exceptional:

> Dr Cartwright got one of the students to examine the patient's
> cardiovascular system. The student began to do so....
> Meanwhile the doctor asked James Bury to come round and look
> at the patient. Bury said he thought the patient's face and
> neck looked 'rather red'.
> Dr Cartwright queried this, and Bury changed his answer to
> 'yellow'.
> Dr Cartwright called over another of the students and asked
> for his opinion on the patient's colouring. He replied he
> would say the patient was 'well tanned'.
> Dr Cartwright agreed, and wrote 'well tanned' on the
> blackboard.

The recognition of abnormal signs - or at least signs that are
potentially abnormal - is therefore something which students certainly
have to learn in many instances. They find themselves unsure how to
produce competent descriptions of what they see, hear and feel.
Sometimes the required perceptions escape them altogether. On one
occasion I was with a group in a medical unit. The consultant was
talking about 'cyanosis' - a bluish tinge to the face associated with
heart disorders. The patient we were discussing did not, he said,
exhibit cyanosis, and that made him suspect that she had not had a
heart attack. For the sake of comparison he ushered us across the ward
to look at another patient. This woman, he maintained, did have
cyanosis, and therefore was much more likely to have had a myocardiac
infarction. Looking at the patient, the students were quite clearly
puzzled, and they confessed themselves unable to detect the bluish
tinge to the complexion that the consultant was drawing attention to.

Sometimes, of course, the problems of 'seeing' are those of novel
technology. Students, for instance, are not familiar with peering
through instruments like opthalmoscopes, and consequently have great
difficulty in discovering the appropriate signs. Similarly, they are
unaccustomed to interpreting the 'objective' findings of X-ray plates.
Although in this context, too, it is not simply a matter of
interpreting observations which are 'obvious', and immediately

apparent to all. Students often simply do not see what they should see, let alone appreciate the significance of such observations.

Even the apparently 'concrete' perception of physical contact - palpation - can be equally elusive. For instance, during a surgical session a consultant was demonstrating a swelling in a female patient's neck:

> So here is this swelling in her neck, and there is no doubt about the state of this - no doubt about her thyroid state.

> The consultant got one of the girl students to come and examine the thyroid. She did so and reported her findings to us, 'There is a soft swelling - with soft edges - not nodules'.

> The surgeon replied, 'I thought it was nodular myself'.

> 'I couldn't find any nodules'. She palpated the patient's neck once more, 'No, I can't find any nodules (hesitantly).

> 'You're hedging. Let's get another opinion'. The surgeon asked a second student to come and examine the patient.

> 'It feels quite smooth in the right lobe, but in the isthmus there might be a discrete lump. But otherwise I agree....'

> The surgeon made no immediate comment, but when the patient had gone back to her bed in the ward, he said that we would see who was right tomorrow, when he operated on the patient. He told the students to be sure to see a specimen of the patient's gland.

In the event, when the operation was carried out the surgeon maintained that the thyroid was in fact quite clearly nodular, and that his perception was unquestionably justified.

On occasion students were asked to produce drawings to illustrate their findings - to indicate the pattern of a pulse, or to indicate the position and size of organs, lumps and so on. Such drawings, as often as not, demonstrated aptly the range of different perceptions which had been made.

The various examples I have provided illustrate the various problems students encounter in producing competent descriptions of clinical phenomena. In the course of bedside teaching students are routinely required to 'observe', 'notice', 'make use of the common senses', 'use your eyes', and so on. The patient is treated as a field, open to inspection, which will yield, objectively, the signs which index underlying pathology. But inexperienced students are often unable to perceive such observable 'facts'. On the contrary, they must learn how to see, hear, feel and smell. While they can produce descriptions of some sort - as anyone could - 'correct' perceptions are not immediately given to their consciousness.

The students' inability to produce competent descriptions was sometimes the occasion for fairly scathing remarks from clinicians (as with the boys who were variously called 'buffoon' and 'moron'). The doctors' exasperated comments are reminiscent of Don Juan's supposed

responses to Castaneda, and Silverman (1975) has recently drawn
attention to this aspect of Castaneda's account of his education at the
hands of the Yaqui magician. Silverman points out how the texts reveal
the problems faced by anyone who is learning - or attempting to learn -
the world and himself from within another's frame of reference. Castaneda's problem always seems to be this: in seeking to understand his
alien, novel experiences he is never sure as to what it is that he is
'meant' to experience. (For instance, he is told to discover his 'spot',
the place where he feels most at ease. Yet he has no available method
for discovering where his spot might be. When he is informed that he
has now found his spot, he still has no idea how he found it or what is
so special about it). Since his groping inquiries are doomed to be
inappropriate, his teacher is suitably derisive and exasperated.

Clinical teachers are clearly more forthcoming than cryptic Yaqui
Indian magicians (real or imagined). But in both contexts, the basic
problem is the same. The teacher cannot 'have' the experience for the
student. He or she can tell the students when they are 'right' or
'wrong', and when they are 'getting warmer'. But there is no way of
guaranteeing that students will automatically hear, see or feel in
precisely the same way as does a teacher. There are no rules that
guarantee it, over and above the basic requirement of argued techniques
and reliable technology. Ultimately all the teacher can do is to say
'Hear it this way', 'Feel it soft' and so on.

However, in observing the 'objective' features of diagnostic signs,
students have to learn the distinctive ways of perceiving. The
consensus of such perceptions - which will warrant their status as
'objective facts' - is provided by the shared 'grammar' of perception
which is shared by the community of practitioners who mutually recognise
each other as competent. Frequently students have trouble in producing
competent descriptions until after they have been told what they should
have perceived, when, perhaps, they return to have a second or third
try.

If students have trouble in producing descriptions of 'signs', then
they have equal, if not greater difficulty in eliciting and formulating
symptoms. By their very nature many symptoms are hard to describe
adequately. Patients and medical personnel do not necessarily have a
shared language in which to share the personal feelings of pain, nausea,
discomfort and so on. Pain, in particular, demands that students learn
to manipulate a range of different descriptive labels which are assumed
to constitute a common language between professionals and laypersons
(e.g. a 'stabbing pain', a 'dull ache', a 'crushing pain'). One
clinician I observed suggested too that they could sometimes try
attaching colour labels - an angry red pain, a dull grey ache and so on.
On other occasions students were encouraged to look for nonverbal clues
which might accompany patients' descriptions of their symptoms. Hand
gestures are often held to be very revealing. The characteristic
'crushing' chest pain associated with a heart attack is quite often
accompanied by a clenching of the fist when patients attempt to describe
it. The sharp, stabbing pain, of say, a gastric ulcer is
characteristically indicated by a more localised indication - the
patient often pointing with a finger at one particular spot. One
patient was searching for an appropriate description of his symptom,
while rubbing his chest: the clinician 'read' the gesture as indicating
'heartburn'. Similarly, students are taught to interpret patients'

posture, expression, gait and so on.

If patients are ambulatory, for instance, students are urged to
observe the way they walk, as gait may be indicative of balance,
coordination and specific motor disorders. For instance:

Dr Maxwell asked Jameson for possible signs of vitamin
deficiency. 'Weight loss', he replied.
'I'll let him off with that', said Dr Maxwell. He turned
to Graham Kennedy,
'Tongue....'
Dr Maxwell retorted immediately 'Legs', asking the others
'Which is more important, his tongue or my legs?'
This was followed by blank looks and silence from all the
students.
Dr Maxwell then jumped up and walked off (much to our
surprise). He then called to us to pull open the curtains
round the bed, and watch him. Dr Maxwell then limped back
to the bedside, imitating the characteristic gait of a
person with a drop-foot.

When patients are sitting up in bed, too, students are urged to observe
them: if they are sitting propped up on a number of pillows, this may
indicate 'orthopnoea' - that is, sitting or lying propped up to ease
difficult breathing.

Throughout this sort of diagnostic activity students find themselves
attempting to perceive the 'right' things, interpret them adequately
and piece them together in order to formulate adequate 'diagnoses'. In
some instances they are urged to generate diagnoses on the basis just
of particular observations, in snap 'end of the bed' diagnoses. In
other instances they have to piece together a more complex semiological
field in order to induce an underlying pattern. The 'detective work'
depends upon students' ability to arrange the various manifestations
into a coherent pattern. Individual 'signs' and 'symptoms' gain their
significance insofar as they can be located within a particular Gestalt.

The patterning, and the predictability of bedside findings is often
referred to in relation to 'classic' cases and 'classic' clinical
pictures. For instance, in relation to heart sounds, a senior
registrar summarised a patient in this manner.

'She's got mitral stenosis, this woman. She's got
absolutely classic signs of mitral stenoses. Don't worry
too much if you didn't hear it....I think she'll be gone
(discharged) on Monday I'm afraid.

The doctor's regret suggested that they would be losing a particularly
'good' example, and that students would have little chance of returning
to listen to the patient's chest once more. Similarly, in the context
of interpreting X-rays of the small bowel, a surgeon remarked, 'If you
saw this patient, you might see the classic step-ladder effect'. That
is, a visible and palpable 'corrugated' effect in the abdomen.

The description of pain - in this instance its location - illustrates
this as well. A student was taking a history from a middle aged woman:

Anne asked, 'We know you had some pain: where was it?'
The patient indicated a spot. 'Just here. You can put
your finger on it'. She indicated the spot by digging
in her index finger.
Mr Fuller turned to the other students and asked them
where that was. One volunteered the answer, 'The
epigastrium'. The surgeon asked for a more precise
definition.
'Just right of the mid line, the student suggested.
Mr Fuller looked at the patient's tummy, 'Just about
mid line, I'd say. Visceral pain always occurs in the
mid line. It's pretty classic. Fore gut pain occurs
in the epigastrium, mid gut pain occurs in the umbilical
area, lower gut pain in the lower abdomen....'

Here the surgeon appeared to be insisting that the location of the
referred pain, which appeared to the students (and to me) to be to the
right, fitted the 'classic' picture, while he filled out and elaborated
that classic pattern.

In these various ways, then, students are not merely required to
'notice' and remark upon isolated phenomena. Such manifestations are
held to make sense - indeed, are worthy of note - only in the context
of a Gestalt. By and large, the 'signs' and 'symptoms' add up to a
significant picture in the context of some overall pattern - a pattern,
moreover, which can be matched to some well established 'type' of
disease.

NORMAL ILLNESS

Hitherto I have argued that bedside teaching is an organised way for the
display of clinical methods in reproducing the relevant clinical 'facts
of the case'. At this point I shall consider the nature of a 'case'.
The 'documentary method' (Garfinkel, 1967) that doctors and medical
students employ is a twofold process. There are two levels of
interpretation involved in the production of diagnoses: they are
closely and dialectically related. In the first instance it is the
task of medical investigators to treat 'signs' and 'symptoms' as
indexing underlying physiological conditions. Though not always
successful, they try to relate these indices in order to read off a
coherent diagnosis, indicating the presence of an identifiable illness,
disorder or syndrome. At the second level, the patient's condition is
itself an 'index' or a 'case' of the disease in question. Just as the
separate and individual signs in the particular patient are understood
in the light of what is known about the typical onset and course of the
illness under normal circumstances.

For the purposes of clinical education, then, the exercise does not
simply consist in the observation and diagnosis of the patient's
presenting complaint. It should also provide occasion for students to
learn about 'the disease' in question, and related conditions. That is,
'normal illness' is invoked.

By using the term 'normal illness' I deliberately parallel the notion
of 'normal crimes' (Sudnow, 1965). Sudnow describes how American Public
Defendants (PDs) come to construct typologies of offences and the people

most likely to commit them. As Sudnow puts it:

> He learns to speak knowledgeably of 'burglars', 'petty
> theives', 'drunks', 'rapists', 'narcos' etc., and to
> attribute to them personal biographies, modes of usual
> criminal activity, criminal histories, psychological
> characteristics, and social backgrounds.

Similarly, the PD constructs an ecological understanding of offences -
that is a sense of where crimes are likely to occur. Hence, what
Sudnow calls 'normal crimes' are

> those occurrences whose typical features, e.g., the ways
> they usually occur and the characteristics of persons
> who commit them (as well as the typical victims and
> typical scenes), are known and attended to by the PD.
> For any of a series of offense types the PD can provide
> some form of proverbial characterization.

Thus the relationship between 'the facts of the case' and what is
'normal' is an important practical problem for the public defendant, and
on his interpretation rests the treatment of the case.

   The medical practitioner is likewise engaged in matching the observed
characteristics of a presenting case to 'normal illnesses'. On the
determination of the normal illness involved depends the expected course
and outcome of the disorder and the treatment of choice. This can be
illustrated in the following report of a teaching period, during which
the physician in charge attempted to demonstrate that the patient
displayed the features of 'normal' illness.

> Dr Mayo took us downstairs to the women's ward: he led
> us into the teaching room and sent two 'strong men' to go
> and bring in the patient's bed from the ward....

> Dr Mayo then went and brought the patient himself. As
> she came in he told us that he had interrupted her
> physiotherapy to bring her to be taught on.

> The patient sat up on the bed, and we all got chairs and
> sat round the bed. 'Who don't we pick on?' asked Dr Mayo,
> looking round the group of students - and decided to ask
> Hilary Morris to begin by taking a history.

> The patient interjected that she had told her story so
> often that, 'I should have brought along a tape recording'.
> (She did not however seem to resent participating in the
> teaching session, and was very cheerful). Hilary asked
> her what had made her first come into hospital.

> 'I'll start right from the beginning' the patient began,
> and Hilary encouraged her to do so.

> The patient described how she had woken up one morning
> with a badly swollen toe-joint, which was very painful.

> Dr Mayo quickly broke in and asked Watson if this rang and
> bells for him: Watson prevaricated, and said there were
> 'several possibilities'. Finally he suggested gout. 'What
> causes gout?' asked Dr Mayo. Watson replied, 'Formerly it

was port'. 'Do you really believe that?'. Watson remained
silent, looked puzzled. Carpenter said it was mostly caused
by drugs. Dr Mayo agreed that it was 'iatrogenic'. He
described briefly that modern diuretics (which, he added, one
uses a lot) lead to accumulations of uric acid. Watson
interrupted and asked what was exchanged for the uric acid.
Dr Mayo said he wasn't sure: he suggested that for next
Monday Watson read up on the effects of diuretics.

The patient then continued her story, and went on to say that
her family doctor had told her it was 'a case for the
orthopaedic'. Amongst other things 'the orthopaedic' said
they could cut out the joint, but she had said 'I'll let well
alone and keep my joint'.

The patient had then developed a 'tingling', and pain in her
right hand: she had previously caught that hand in a door,
and she thought the discomfort might be connected with that.
She said that the tingling condition in her hand had been
diagnosed as 'something internal' - and she added, she was
sorry, she couldn't remember more accurately than that.

Dr Mayo turned to the students and asked them to 'translate'
what she had been trying to say. One of the students
volunteered that it might be 'carpal tunnel syndrome'.

Dr Mayo summarised this condition briefly. Watson jumped in
with an objection to his description - 'Isn't it usually the
median nerve?' Dr Mayo looked slightly annoyed and pointed
out that he had corrected himself when he had said it was
the ulnar nerve, and had said it was the median the second
time.

Dr Mayo said to the patient, 'You had trouble with your
shoulder too, didn't you?', and she agreed that she had had
trouble. All this time Dr Mayo had the patient's case notes
with him and he constantly referred to them in bringing out
the patient's history.

The patient also volunteered that she now had a painful and
swollen knee. Dr Mayo commented that the hand might have
been blamed on something else, but now we had a shoulder
and a knee as well, 'We definitely have a polyarthritis'. It
was, he added, 'a very typical story'.

The patient volunteered that she gained relief in her hands
by soaking them in hot water, and Dr Mayo commented to
Hilary Morris, 'This is the basis of the therapy, isn't it?'
'Hmmmm' (nodding).

'What is it?' Dr Mayo continued. But Hilary in fact
appeared not to know. There was no response from any of the
others in the group, and Dr Mayo told them that the
treatment was with hot paraffin wax - which he described
briefly.

Dr Mayo summed up some aspects of the case, and in doing so
made a mistake in the timing of the history - her visit to
the orthopaedic specialists. The patient corrected him.
'Sorry, I've got the story wrong', and Dr Mayo hastily
referred to the case notes to correct his summary.

Dr Mayo then turned to the students, 'What are you thinking of?'

Hilary Morris - 'Nothing'.

'Well, what diseases of the joints do you know?'

'Rheumatoid arthritis', Hilary suggested.

Another of the students offered 'Osteoarthritis', but added that he wasn't sure of the difference between osteoarthritis and rheumatoid arthritis, as he'd never seen a case of osteoarthritis.

Dr Mayo then wrote the following schema on the blackboard:

	Osteo	Rheumatoid
Age	60+	40+
Sex	=	30 : 10
Joints	Big	Hand/small
General condition	Well	Unwell

Dr Mayo then read off the patient's history against these categories. 'As for age' he began, 'the patient said she was 53, she's equal on that'.

'That's me being difficult', put in the patient.

When it came to sex and the joints affected, Dr Mayo said that rheumatoid arthritis seemed to be indicated.

When it came to the final category - the patient's general health, the pattern seemed less clear. 'When you came in, you said you hadn't been feeling well, and had been losing your appetite'. The patient replied that she hadn't felt unwell. Dr Mayo persisted, and said that she had been sweating rather: she countered that she had had sweats for many years past. Dr Mayo said she had had a poor appetite, and the patient replied that she had 'never been a big eater'.

Dr Mayo, leaving the patient protesting once more that she hadn't felt ill, and hadn't had any headaches or anything.... Dr Mayo referred to the case notes: 'In fact she had a pyrexia when she came in - a spiky temperature....'

Dr Mayo then went on to a discussion of a number of haematological points, and he said that the presence of a changed ESR 'would be nice'.

Dr Mayo and the students went on to examine the patient's right knee, which had been swollen and painful according to her history. Dr Mayo asked Carpenter to tell us what he saw. He immediately started to palpate the knee: Dr Mayo told him - gently and in a pleasant tone of voice - that he had told him to tell us what he saw.
....

When Carpenter did come to palpate the knee, Dr Muir asked him if he could detect any fluid in the knee, and Carnie replied that he didn't know how to test for fluid. Dr Mayo explained how to squeeze the region of the patella, and then try to bounce the patella up and down on the bone underneath, when one gets the sensation of fluid underneath. However,

when he tried to do it himself, he was unable to produce the
right effect. 'That's me being awkward again', said the
patient, with a rather satisfied little smile.

This extended summary illustrates a number of features involved in
assembling the diagnosis. Throughout the interaction the clinician who
was conducting the teaching made reference to the normal features of the
case. Indeed, his first summary of the patient's history was that it
was 'a very typical story'. The patient herself, on the other hand,
seemed to orient herself to the particularity of her case - or so I
interpret her rather self-satisfied interjections on her being 'awkward'
when she appeared not to 'fit' the doctor's classifications. This is an
example of how, in producing 'normal crimes' and 'normal illnesses',
practitioners proceed by discounting the particularities and
idiosyncracies of the case in the course of formulating its typicality.

This aspect of the physician's work in defining the patient as a
typical case of rheumatoid arthritis can be seen in his simple
classification of osteo- and rheumatoid arthritis. This schematic
device presented a series of decision rules for distinguishing between
the normal onset and presentation of the two illnesses. Yet the
implementation of these decisions in practice turned out to be
problematic.

In the course of clinical teaching there is a constant tension between
definitions of 'normal' illness and the particularities of individual
patients' presenting complaints. Students need to be able to learn the
typical course and appearance of any given illness, despite deviations
from the normal in patients they see. Clinicians therefore make
repeated references to possible mis-matches between 'text book'
descriptions of illnesses and their presentation.

For instance, during one period of medical teaching, I noted the
following sequence of comments which illustrate the use of 'typical'
formulations as a device for generating 'normal' expectations, and
distinctions between type and presenting case.

Dr.   He's as hyperthyroid as they come...what in his
       history is not quite typical - about his weight loss?
       (Pause - no reply from the students). His appetite
       should be increased - in fact he's off his food.
....

Dr.   What about the CVS - what would you expect there?

St.   Tachycardia - bounding rhythm

Dr.   What rhythm could you sometimes get?

St.   Galloping rhythm

Dr.   Well, you could

St.   Atrial fibrillation....
....

Dr.   Now in severe thyrotoxicosis - I've never seen it -
       but there are two signs that the text books give.
       There's thyroid acropathy - it's like finger clubbing.
       You'd need to be in an endocrinology unit to see it....

106

Here the physician's reference to a 'typical' indication of the
illness that is not present in the case in question is parallelled by
his closing reference to 'text book' signs which are not routinely
present in many cases. In both instances the clinician alerts the
students to the problematic nature of the relationships between
typifications and instances of illness. In both instances, the
students need to 'go beyond' the indications of concrete presentations
to read into them the indications of normal presentations. It is the
availability of such typifications that informs a wide range of teaching
exchanges at the bedside.

The obverse of the treatment of 'normal' illness and textbook
knowledge is the contingency that these typifications may fail to
include items of practical use in concrete contexts of diagnosis and
treatment. In the following extract, a physician comments on the gap
between 'theory' and practice in the context of cardiology. He had
asked the students to draw diagrams illustrating the 'classic' heart
sounds associated with various forms of impairment of the heart. In the
teaching room the physician went through the diagrams that the students
had produced.

> Dr Maxwell began, 'Right, mitral incompetence'. He went over
> to one of the students, 'What have you drawn? Let me see.
> First heart sound....Yes, reduced heart sound', (he draws on
> the board). 'True or false?' The books are wrong. Every
> book I've seen draws a murmur to the second sound and stops
> it there. The great thing about mitral incompetence is...
> the second sound is buried in the murmur.

The contrast between 'text book' rules and rules in use in the context
of clinical teaching can be indicated by reference to the notion of
'routine'. 'Routine' is an important organising principle in teaching
and learning clinical procedures. The elicitation of a history and its
documentation, and the performance of a physical examination of a
patient should, students are told, be done according to a well worked
out 'routine'. That is, it should be done systematically and
methodically, following a number of steps in sequence.

Yet it is clear that investigations of inordinate length are not the
normal state of affairs that competent doctors acknowledge as correct.
While such an approach might be defensible as 'painstaking', it is not
normally a practical way of setting about getting clinical work done.
Time is not available for such methods to be worked through completely
in all cases. The experienced worker demonstrates ability and
competence by producing a history and examination in a way which does
not conform to a literal adherence to the routine. Students are
therefore confronted with two aspects of practical rule use: that the
symptoms must be mastered and followed, but also that experienced
following of the rules implies an apparent 'breaking' of the rules.
The routine is, in the last analysis, 'honoured in the breach' by the
'experienced' practitioner.

Clinicians present the students with this dual nature of clinical
procedure.

> The patient was an old man of seventy who was suffering from
> severe myocardial failure. Dr Shaw elicited a history from

him for our benefit. The patient had been a road crossing
'lollipop man'....He had come into hospital this time because
he was suffering a severe pain in his chest. Dr Shaw
questioned him further about the pain, and any other symptoms
....Dr Shaw probed with further questions about the pain -
had it moved into the neck or arm? The old man reported
that it had not moved.
....

Asked for his previous history, the patient said that the
only other illness he had had was when he had come into
hospital that January: he had had pain in his calves, and he
told us that this had been a 'coronary thrombosis'. Dr Shaw
did not follow this up at the time.
....

During the course of the history, Dr Shaw stopped and
realised that he had not demonstrated getting basic
information - the patient's name, age and so on. He then
produced the patient's charts from the foot of the bed and
read off some of the basic facts about the patient.
....

After further questioning the patient, Dr Shaw took us
outside and we stood in the corridor. One of the students
pointed out that Dr Shaw had forgotten to ask if there has
been any oedema. The doctor agreed that he had forgotten
that. Dr Shaw then referred to the January admission. The
patient had told us today that he had had a coronary
thrombosis which had been a 'pain in his leg'. In fact,Dr
Shaw told us, the old man had had a severe cardiac failure
and had 'died'; but he had no memory of his previous attack,
apart from pain in the hardened arteries in his leg. Dr Shaw
pointed out that he had not wanted to remind the patient of
that, or let him know that he had died on that occasion.

In passing, this extract further illustrates two aspects already
alluded to: the preservation of 'closed awareness', and the clinician's
invocation of 'in fact' clauses in reconstructing the patient's history.
It also illustrates how a physician may not stick slavishly to the
systematic, sequential ordering of history taking, as specified in
'official' rubrics. Indeed, after the particular session, the students
themselves referred to this. They remarked the contrast between what
they had just witnessed and the advice they had themselves been given
in introductory lectures on clinical method. They expressed
disappointment that Dr Shaw had been 'so unsystematic' in his approach
to the patient.

INDETERMINATION AND TECHNICALITY

Hitherto I have been trying to indicate how clinical work is organised
according to two complementary principles. On the one hand, the
construction of teaching encounters can be seen as a device for the
reproduction of knowledge of which the students and the clinicians can
be sure and certain: that is, the reproduction of warranted clinical
'facts'. On the other hand, the production of such factual accounts
depends upon personal 'experience' in interpreting the rules of clinical

procedure. These twin aspects of the production and reproduction of medical knowledge have been examined by Jamous and Peloille (1970), who apply the two principles in a general account of occupations - based upon what they term the ratio between Indetermination and Technicality (abbreviated to I/T) (see also Atkinson, Reid and Sheldrake, 1977).

By 'Technicality' is meant those aspects of professional work which are susceptible to codification in terms of explicit, public rules, procedures and techniques. The 'technical' aspects of professional work are those procedures which can (at least, hypothetically) be expressed in a precise list of unambiguous specifications. 'Indetermination', on the other hand, refers to those varieties of 'tacit' and private knowledge which are not susceptible to such specification. It is not made explicit, and remains untranslatable into precisely formulated rules or prescriptions.

There is therefore a difference between the mode of transmission of such types of knowledge, and in the relationship of the worker (or teacher) to the knowledge itself. In the case of 'technical' modes of knowledge, transmission could be based upon 'mechanical' reproduction, unaltered from generation to generation and from place to place. The sole criterion for success would be complete mastery of the relevant techniques, on the basis of rote learning, locomotor coordination and so on. Such cultural reproduction could be achieved in a completely 'impersonal' way. The transmission of 'indeterminate' means of production and knowledge would depend upon 'example', and the observation of a practitioner by the trainee. The novice would have to 'pick up' such knowledge rather than being taught it explicitly. Whereas 'technical' expertise could be defined in terms of public and impersonal criteria, 'indeterminate' expertise would depend upon less readily definable and accountable criteria. In Jamous and Peloille's terminology, indeterminate knowledge thus becomes located in personal attributes (or 'virtualities') of the producer himself - who is thus an 'owner' of the means of production and reproduction, rather than simply a user of them.

Now Jamous and Peloille do not claim that occupations can be classified or understood simply in terms of indetermination or technicality alone. Rather they argue that occupations are marked by a mixture of explicit and implicit expertise, by publicly available techniques and private 'rules of thumb'. What they employ is the ratio of Technicality to Indetermination as a device for the classification and understanding of occupations and their work. They express the core of their argument in this way:

> The I/T ratio expressed the possibility of transmitting by means of apprenticeship, the mastery of intellectual or material instruments and to achieve a given result. This makes it possible to appreciate the limits of this transmissibility; i.e., the part played in the production process by 'means' that can be mastered in the form of rules (T), in proportion to the means that escape rules and, at a given historical moment, are attributed to virtualities of producers (I).

Although Jamous and Peloille begin their argument by setting aside any 'absolutist' definition of the 'professions' (e.g., such as 'trait' theories), implicitly, they use the I/T ratio to reintroduce 'the professions' in a somewhat different guise:

> The occupations and activities which concern us are the ones which lie on that sector of the dimension where the I/Ts are usually high. This sector does not include all occupations nor only the occupations usually called 'professions'.

Nevertheless, they confine their remarks to 'professions' and do not indicate what other occupations might fall on this 'sector'; it is also implied that a high I/T ratio is a common attribute of those occupations normally designated 'professional'.

There are a number of shortcomings in the approach advocated by Jamous and Peloille. They are highly ambivalent as to whether the indetermination and technicality to which they refer are to be seen as 'objective' attributes of an occupational group and their work, or whether they constitute claims professed by occupational groups - that is, they are occupational ideologies.

The central problem in Jamous and Peloille's use of the I/T ratio can be highlighted by reference to my previous comments on competent rule use. They are in error in trying to separate out the two aspects; all rule use implies an interpretation ability on the part of the rule user, and such interpretive competence is not spelled out in the formulation of the rules itself (cf. Bittner, 1965; Zimmerman, 1970; Emmerson and Pollner, 1978). However much the rules of procedure may be codified, the concrete application of the spirit of the rules depends upon 'tacit' understandings. What we refer to as a 'knack' or 'flair' or 'experience' refers to such competence in the application of interpretive procedures in the production and reproduction of knowledge. Hence Jamous and Peloille's dichotomy is a false one: what they treat as two independent factors in their I/T ratio are inextricably intertwined.

On the other hand, it is possible that the notions of indetermination and technicality constitute a rhetoric in which are couched claims concerning professional work and expertise. From this point of view one might inspect how varieties of knowledge are warranted by practitioners by reference to the two principles of production and reproduction.

The language of indetermination is a language of personal knowledge. The language of 'experience' is the common currency of a stratified and segmented occupation. It is congruent with segmentation since it relies on differences in personal experience, the distinctiveness of concrete occasions, of practice and the diversity of individual careers. 'Tacit' knowledge depends upon the consensus of discrete groups with shared occupational ideologies and biographies. The rhetoric of 'experience' is also that of a stratified occupation. It emphasises a view of socialisation and expertise founded upon a lengthy period of induction in the 'mysteries' and arcane knowledge of the occupation: the accumulation of relevant experience is to be gained painstakingly in the course of a practitioner's unfolding career. Hence expertise is only to be guaranteed by seniority and length of 'experience'. However well-informed a young practitioner, and whatever the level of his technical learning, it still requires the accumulation of 'experience' to transform him into a fully competent practitioner. As Jamous and

Peloille themselves emphasise, the 'apprenticeship' approach to
socialisation, and its reliance upon an apostolic transmission of
knowledge from practitioner to apprentice, is predicated on the
congruence between the stratification and segmentation of the
profession. If the rhetoric of technicality is expressive of the
common knowledge, and publicly accountable knowledge base of the
profession, then that of 'indetermination' ensures the non
accountability and autonomy of the profession, and of segments within
it.

In the course of clinical teaching, appeal is often made to
'experience', and 'judgement'. Such knowledge is treated as personal
and therefore as less technical or determinate, than the prescriptions
of 'science' and the formulations of text books. In contrast to the
context free, universalistic connotations of 'science', experience is
a personal matter, dependent on the biography of the clinician. The
quality of 'experience' gained depends, for example, on where one is
trained and practised, with whom one has been a doctor, and when. In
the course of his career, the competent clinician amasses a stock of
relevant experience, upon which he can draw.

The following extracts from my field notes illustrate how clinicians
may make appeals to experience in decision making on diagnosis and
patient management. For instance, in the first extract, the teaching
physician alerts the students to personal experience in therapy - and
how the locale of one's treatment and practice is a major factor in
clinicians' adoption of therapeutic measures.

> They discussed the problems of high blood pressure and
> reducing it. Dr Cowan told us that on admission, the
> patient had a palpable fourth heart sound, and they had
> been afraid he'd go into failure. 'The question is', he
> said, 'What drug do you use to reduce blood pressure?'
> The students suggested a number of possible treatments,
> and Dr Cowan commented, 'You get used to one drug.
> Propranadol is used a lot in Edinburgh'.

The same consideration is apparent in the consultant surgeon's
pronouncement in the following extract. The remarks were noted in a
tutorial class on breast cancer. The surgeon had explained to the
clinique the difference between 'simple' and 'radical' mastectomies.
Returning to the patient who had provided the starting point for the
more general discussion, the surgeon told us,

> 'In this city, she'd have a simple mastectomy; in
> Edinburgh it's accepted that most units do a simple
> mastectomy....'

In both of these illustrations, then, appeal is made to 'Edinburgh' in
recommending choices of treatment. 'The way things are done here' is
a common enough appeal to local experience and ideology in most
processes of socialisation, including socialisation into organisations
and occupational groups. In the second example, the surgeon also draws
attention to a further dimension of segmentation: 'most' units do a
simple mastectomy, but it is not a categorical statment, and there is
the possibility of differences in approach between units within the

same city. The autonomy of practitioners allows for the development of different treatments of choice in different sectors of the same medical school.

Pharmacology is a topic where 'experience' is frequently drawn on in justifying or condemning the use of particular drugs or dosages. In the following field note, the physician refers to fashion and personal experience in decision making in this field.

> The clinique then proceeded to a discussion of therapy. Dr Mayo asked what drugs you would use to treat rheumatoid arthritis. Tim Watson replied, 'Anti-inflammatory drugs - aspirin'. Dr Mayo agreed that aspirin was still the best treatment, provided it relieves the pain sufficiently. He went on to comment on some other drugs which were, as he put it, 'in vogue', but which can produce unpleasant side effects.
>
> Dr Mayo went on to comment that one needs to monitor blood levels: in aspirin the upper limit of dosage was indicated by the patient's experiencing 'ringing in the ears'. He pointed out that it was not always possible to get blood levels monitored, and so you have to 'use your own judgement'. And, he added, 'you need to use drugs you are used to'.

The 'empirical' basis of some therapeutic procedures is frequently repeated, and contrasted with the claims of 'scientific' knowledge. This is again illustrated in the following case, where the 'do or die' aspect of the treatment offered threw into relief the practical need for action, in contrast to the niceties of 'theoretical' pharmacology.

Similarly, in the following extract, the physician refers to the possibilities of action by the _ad hoc_ use of therapeutic techniques, as a possible departure from established procedure.

> Dr Rosen took us back to the teaching room, and told us that the patient we had just seen had multiple myeloma. He told us that there was no chance of a cure, but that they were about to embark on a course of palliative treatment. There were two drugs that they were going to use, both in fairly massive doses. He said that they were advised to treat patients of this sort for one month on the drugs, and one month off - to give the bone marrow a chance to recuperate. However, he added, they might find it better to administer the drugs one week on and one week off, or two weeks and two weeks respectively. 'One has to play it be ear', he concluded.

The warrant of 'experience' is often referred to as a source of certainty or trust in the face of the vagaries of fashion and novelty. This too can be illustrated from the field of pharmaceuticals. Since the 'therapeutic revolution' in the 1930s, the number of different pharmaceutical preparations has increased exponentially (Norton, 1969). Doctors are being introduced to a vast range of medications for illnesses of all sorts. Many of the preparations that are taken up and widely used gain their popularity partly on the basis of 'fashion' (cf.

112

Coleman et al., 1966). Whilst 'fashion' and 'experience' can both be contrasted to 'science' they are also themselves contrasted. The dictates of 'fashion' remain untried by the warrant of 'science' (e.g., controlled trials over a long period) or of carefully amassed personal experience in clinical practice.

The importance of 'experience' and personal knowledge has been noted before. Becker and other authors of *Boys in White* note the importance of 'experience' to students and teachers alike. They identify a group perspective based upon this action, and they take the 'clinical experience perspective' to refer to 'actual experience in dealing with patients and disease....' As they comment, it is often used to contrast with 'theoretical' and 'scientific' knowledge:

> ...even though it substitutes for scientifically certified knowledge, it can be used to legitimate a choice of procedures for a patient's treatment and can even be used to rule out use of some procedures that have been scientifically established. (Becker et al., 1961, p.225).

This important place that is reserved for 'experience' has often been linked with the constellation of factors referred to as 'uncertainty'. Freidson (1970) provides a classic formulation. He summarises the Kansas evidence, and then continues,

> ...the practitioner is very prone to emphasise the idea of indeterminacy or uncertainty, not the idea of regularity or of lawful, scientific behaviour. Whether or not that idea faithfully represents actual deficiencies in available knowledge or technique it does provide the practitioner with a psychological ground from which to justify his pragmatic emphasis on first hand experience.

Here Freidson emphasises uncertainty of knowledge, suggesting that personal knowledge and experience are to be contrasted with notions of regularity and predictability. He also tends to account for this at the level of the psychology of the individual practitioner. Fox (1957) takes a similar view in her discussion of 'training for uncertainty'. Like Freidson, she tends to treat it as a psychological problem that medical students need to come to terms with. I have already suggested one way in which such formulations may be inadequate. The idea of 'uncertainty' or 'indetermination' needs to be seen not simply as the outcome of individual psychology, but must also be seen in the context of professional segmentation, and as a reflection of the conditions of autonomy on the part of practitioners. Further, in both the formulations of the 'clinical mentality' referred to above, the theme of 'training for uncertainty' has been over-stressed. 'Training for dogmatism' has been almost entirely overlooked.

'Dogmatism' is by no means the opposite of personal knowledge; it is part and parcel of the same view of personal 'experience'. The clinician who appeals to his personal knowledge does so not by reference to his uncertainty, nor the uncertainty of his colleagues. Rather, he bases his actions and decisions on what is taken as a bedrock - the certainty - of direct experience. The appeal to 'experience' is (*pace* Freidson) taken to provide knowledge of regularity and stability. The clinician operates in a state of personal certainty, in the sure warrant

of his own personal experience. Hence the appeal to 'experience' is
taken to provide knowledge of regularity and stability; but this order
is taken to be inherent in the phenomena, and open to the 'gaze', rather
than residing in systems of theory and fashion. 'The clinic' is
therefore taken to provide the incontrovertible demonstrations of
reality in direct perception of its regularities. The clinician is not
therefore operating in a state of 'uncertainty', but rather operating on
the 'sure' warrant of his stock of experience. In this way, the
students' exposure to this 'real' world of medicine reproduces the
certainty of personal knowledge.

8 Glossing Medicine

This book has been concerned with aspects of the social construction of reality in the context of one phase of medical education. While no claims can be entered as to the 'typicality' of the particular, concrete details reported here, I do want to suggest that what I have reported reflects fundamental and general features of clinical medicine and medical education. The most important of these is the way in which a particular <u>version</u> of medical work and medical knowledge is reproduced through clinical instruction. This in turn reflects the basic premise of 'clinical experience' itself.

As I have remarked already, 'clinical' phases of training rest on the assumption that the trainee is to gain 'practical' knowledge and experience through some form of exposure to, immersion in, and some sort of 'practice' on 'real' settings. Medical education provides the type case of professional training of this sort; the designation 'clinical' has been transposed from medical settings to other occupational contexts. (It has, for instance, been applied to recent developments in legal education. See Rees, 1975).

Throughout this short monograph I have attempted to document, on the basis of my own fieldwork, how this clinical 'reality' is socially organised, achieved and managed. I have therefore provided a detailed account of how a particular sort of medical reality is produced and reproduced. No attempt has been made, therefore, to account for all aspects of undergraduate medical education, nor even to cover all aspects of everyday life among the fourth year students I observed and talked to. The focus of this book has, deliberately, been more limited than that, and certainly does not aim to be a 'holistic' ethnography. The theme of 'clinical experience' has therefore been the dominant, organising theme of this book. In this conclusion I want briefly to consider the nature of this 'experience'.

As I have shown, I hope, the medical reality to which the beginning student is exposed is by no means straightforward. There is nothing 'natural' about such 'reality'. Like any other it is a matter of social construction. What novitiate students are introduced to, then, is not the practical reality of some essential clinical medicine. Rather, they encounter the dramatic enactment of a particular form or version of medical work. It is through that enactment that the potency of such a version or model of medicine is captured and reproduced. I hope I may have conveyed something of the vivid drama of that reproduction: as I suggested in Chapter 2 the medical students find themselves absorbed and 'seduced' by this highly appealing form of work and understanding.

It is, perhaps, worth reminding the reader once again that the mind boggling methods of 'deduction' expounded by the fictional Sherlock Holmes were taken by Conan Doyle from the real life methods of medical inference. (He must have enjoyed the irony that in his stories it was Dr Watson, the medical man, who always proved too dense to follow the great detective's logic). On numerous occasions during my fieldwork

I was struck by the parallels between the Holmesian approach, and the displays of diagnostic acumen produced by the clinical teachers. I found myself identifying, at least tenatively, a style of teaching I labelled 'thaumaturgical' (wonder working). The patients and medical students would find themselves recruited partly as audience, partly as 'stooges', partly as 'props' in displays of clinical expertise and diagnostic skill. The effects of such displays, and of less dramatic styles of teaching too, is to produce vivid firsthand reconstructions of the logic and rationality of clinical medicine. It is as audience to these performances that the students gain their first clinical experiences.

There is something noteworthy here about the only photograph to accompany that classic *Boys in White*. The picture appears on the original dust jacket. It shows seven male medical students, all looking remarkably similar in their white jackets and trousers. They are sitting in a steeply banked lecture theatre, of a kind used in medical schools from their earliest years to the present day. They all have their eyes fixed on something or someone at the front of the theatre; who or what it is we do not know. But this one photograph stands as a remarkable metonym for the nature of clinical education: the students as audience in a dramatic reconstruction, their 'clinical gaze' fixed on their teachers and patients, and on the signs and symptoms they display, absorbed in the clinical world. The photograph from *Boys in White* does not reveal the object of the students' rapt attention: in that book Becker and his colleagues pay but little attention to it. In this monograph I have attempted to follow their gaze, to follow the students' line of vision, and to devote my attention to the drama of clinical instruction.

GLOSSING AND MOCK UPS

Let me begin once more by recapitulating what I take to be the main features of bedside teaching as 'cold medicine'. Student work on patients is managed in such a way that it proceeds 'as if' diagnostic work were starting afresh, although in most cases it is not. 'Cold medicine' (in this sense) is therefore contrived in such a way as to reproduce and parallel what are taken for crucial features of the reality of 'hot medicine'.

What I wish to suggest is that 'cold medicine' is a 'glossing device' (Garfinkel and Sacks, 1970): that is, a device for 'doing observable-reportable understanding'. In other words, bedside teaching practices are socially organised ways by which the actors produce something like a 'working model' of medical diagnosis. Such a model makes observable and teachable the methods whereby diagnosis is normally done by competent members of the medical profession. Garfinkel and Sacks suggest something of the sort in their discussion of glossing practices which they refer to as 'mock-ups': they instance working models as an example:

> *Mock-Ups*. It is possible to buy a plastic engine that will tell something about how auto engines work. The plastic engine preserves certain properties of the auto engine. For example, it will show how the pistons move with respect to the crank shaft; how they are timed to a firing sequence,

an so on....

Let us call that plastic engine an account of an observable
state of affairs. We offer the following observations of
that account's features. First, in the very way that it
provides for an accurate representation of features in the
actual situation, and in the very way it provides for an
accurate representation of some relationships and some
features in the observable situation, it also makes
specifically and deliberately false provision of some of
the <u>essential</u> features of that situation.

(Garfinkel and Sacks, 1970, p.263).

Garfinkel and Sacks' formulation of a 'mock-up' encapsulates precisely
the nature of 'cold medicine' as an account of 'real' medicine, and
providing a model of that state of affairs. In the accomplishment of
such accounting devices, we can see how bedside teaching makes 'accurate
representations' of real medicine (in the methods of history taking,
diagnosis, etc.), and how this is possible since it makes 'specifically
and deliberately false provision of some of the essential features'.
That is, normal clinical methods can be employed insofar as the reality
of previous clinical work is suppressed or held in abeyance for the
duration of the teaching exercise. This feature of bedside interactions
allows for the ways in which it can be controlled and managed by the
'user' (in this case, the teaching clinician). The 'false provision'
(that prior medical work may be discounted) allows for his or her
techniques in managing the transfer of information between the parties,
through prior acquaintance with the patient's condition. Thus the
clinician can 'work' the model and articulate the account.

The cold medicine mock-up can be further illustrated and parallelled
by a brief consideration of recent developments in the teaching of the
natural sciences in secondary schools (cf. Atkinson and Delamont, 1977).
Through the sponsorship of the Nuffield Foundation and the Schools
Council, the past decades have seen major innovations in science
teaching. The main feature of this has been an emphasis upon learning
by 'discovery'. Rather than being the passive recipients of 'facts',
delivered *ex cathedra* by the science teacher, and divorced from their
immediate experience, school pupils should rather learn science by <u>doing</u>
it. That is, they should 'discover' science and scientific
understanding by performing experiments themselves. The teacher's task
became redefined as one of co-ordinating and guiding the pupils' own
'discoveries'.

Now it is by no means the case that the 'discovery' of phenomena in
the natural world can proceed independently from the methods of inquiry
employed in the 'discovery procedure'. As Delamont (1973) has
documented, the classroom practice of such 'mock-ups' of the work of
scientists, requires a great deal of more or less covert 'stage
management' on the part of the teacher. The pupils' line of inquiry
has to be curtailed by the science teacher if they are to 'look for' the
appropriate phenomena, arrive at the 'correct' observation, and hence
'discover' the expected scientific facts.

In this sense, the school science lesson and the bedside teaching
period are similar, in that they both depend for their success on the
teacher's acting 'as if' the answer to the problem were not already

117

known, but needed to be discovered afresh, thus parallelling real
contexts where discovery (scientific or diagnostic) is in fact the
outcome of scientists' or doctors' inquiries.

In both cases, then, the nature of the 'mock-up' depends upon the
'discovery' of appropriate conclusions, by the use of appropriate methods
of inquiry ('experiments' or 'history taking and examination'). In my
discussion of bedside teaching I have explored how 'cold medicine'
provides occasion for the reproduction of clinical and diagnostic
methods. In other words, how the practices of bedside instruction
provide concrete demonstrations of the warranted nature of clinical
knowledge.

WARRANTING KNOWLEDGE

The central concern here is an investigation of how the 'facts of the
case' are determined and legitimated by reference to the procedural
rules of 'correct' and 'methodical' inquiry. When we speak of
ascertaining 'the facts' we assign a special status to certain sorts of
accounts and propositions, as opposed to 'opinions', 'beliefs',
'guesses' and so on; by implication these latter are not granted the
same warrant as well researched, fully documented, correctly retrieved
'facts'. The status of such 'facts' is not something which is inherent
in the accounts of them - but rather resides in the procedures and rules
which are used to establish and validate the knowledge. This is
expressed by McHugh (1970):

> ...nothing - no object, event, or circumstances - determines
> its own status as truth, either to the scientist or to
> science....An event is transformed into the truth only by
> the application of a canon of procedure, a canon that truth-
> seekers use and analysts must formulate as providing the
> possibility of agreement.

The place of such methodic procedures in the determination of 'facts'
is highlighted in Kuhn's analysis of scientific revolutions (Kuhn,
1970). For Kuhn, it is the scientific 'paradigm' which provides the
ground rules for scientists' consensus over appropriate topics for
inquiry, appropriate methods and the sort of answers that might
reasonably be expected. As Kuhn himself puts it, the paradigms

> provide scientists not only with a map but also with the
> directions for map-making. In learning a paradigm the
> scientist acquires theory, methods, and standards
> together, usually in an inextricable mixture.

Kuhn's analysis of 'normal' and 'revolutionary' phases in scientific
research and discovery draws attention to the fact that the practice of
scientific inquiry is inescapably a social activity, insofar as it
depends upon the organised consensus of those engaged in science, and
on their shared methods for the production of scientific knowledge.

The problem of ascertaining and warranting the 'facts of the case' is
by no means confined to natural scientists. It appears as a practical
problem in a wide range of everyday work. This is well documented by
Zimmerman (1966) in his study of case workers in a social welfare

agency.

It is a routine problem for the case workers that they should establish whether applicants are entitled to the money and assistance which they claim. Applicants need to demonstrate 'need', and the agency workers must determine their 'eligibility'. There is, therefore, a crucial distinction between the claimant's 'story' and the 'facts'. For a story to become transferred into a factual account, the case worker must check and validate the 'reliability' of the claimant's account. One important aspect of this process is the way in which case workers rely on documentary evidence. Yet in establishing documentary evidence, 'any old piece of paper' will not do and only 'official' documents will suffice. Such documents are taken to guarantee that the 'facts' that they record have themselves been investigated, processed and recorded in a 'correct' and methodic manner. Bureaucracies and large scale organisations are taken to operate in methodic ways which the case worker recognises as competent in producing 'facts' and 'evidence'.

In the same way, the case worker herself assembles documents on the applicant - producing a 'case' which itself records the case worker's 'investigative stance' of scepticism and methodic inquiry. Thus the case worker assembles the 'facts of the case' in accordance with the legitimate rules of procedure of the bureaucracy, and bases her 'case' on 'evidence' provided by comparable bureaucracies employing equivalent methods of inquiry and documentation. Zimmerman thus points out how workers, whose task it is to produce orderly factual accounts depend upon the demonstrable, rational and methodic ways in which their accounts have been assembled.

A similar perspective is provided by Smith (1973) in her discussion of the production of 'documentary reality', which she describes as 'constituted in those socially organised practices of reporting and accounting, which mediate our relation to "what really happens"'. Smith emphasises how 'the fact' is not what happened in its 'raw', uninterpreted state. The 'factual' resides in the way 'what happened' has been worked up into an account of which itself provides for a 'factual' reading and understanding. The nature of 'factual' accounts, however, allows the reader or hearer to treat them in such a way as to discount its social nature: the organisation of the account is itself 'transparent'. In this context Smith draws a parallel between the social production of facts and the production of commodities. Marx wrote:

> A commodity is...a mysterious thing, simply because in it
> the social character of man's labour appears to them as
> an objective character stamped upon the product of that
> labour.   (Marx, 1954, p.77).

Although such products are created by men's labour, nevertheless they confront their producers as alien objects; the relations between men take on the nature of relations between things (commodities). In much the same way, Smith argues, facts are equally 'mysterious'. They are outcomes of the socially organised ways of dealing with events. Yet they do not appear to be socially produced by men engaged in practical action. On the contrary, we normally employ the notions of 'opinion', 'belief', 'ideology' and 'bias' to locate the social nature of such knowledge; the language of 'fact' excludes the mediation of the social

119

basis of knowledge production.

I wish to consider the practices of bedside teaching in this context
of the production of 'factual' knowledge. 'Cold medicine' should be
seen as a device whereby the rational and methodic nature of clinical
investigation and the retrieval of the 'facts of the case' are
produced and reproduced.

There is a dialectical relationship between 'facts' and the socially
legitimated methods for their 'discovery' and 'testing'. The methodic
nature of their production is a warrant for the 'correctness' of the
facts of the case. At the same time, it is the reliable discovery of
such 'facts' that further furnishes a warrant for the methods of inquiry.
I take it that this is the force of Kuhn's notion of 'normal science',
conducted in accordance with a 'paradigm'. The paradigm provides
approved topics and appropriate research procedures; the successful
accomplishment of such procedures and the 'findings' that are generated
in turn serve to reinforce the value of the paradigm.

In this sense, the accounts of 'facts' are 'reflexive' (Garfinkel,
1967). That is, the accounts of states of affairs are themselves
constitutive of the affairs they describe. As Filmer (1972) paraphrases
Garfinkel,

> rules...are only established as such by their ability to
> organize the settings of practical, everyday, commensense
> actions - an ability which is proven in organising these
> actions.

In the medical context, therefore, the facts of a diagnosis are
guaranteed by the rules and procedures of clinical inquiry which
establish them: by the same token, these procedures are validated
insofar as they generate reproduceable and reportable diagnoses.

Displays of the rational nature of such socially warranted methods are
an important ingredient in a novice's learning of how to become a
competent investigator of facts. Zimmerman (1974) refers to this in his
discussion of welfare agency workers. Those who were new to the job
were instructed by the 'old hands' in the correct application of the
rules of investigative procedure. It was part of their 'on the job'
training that they should adopt a sufficiently sceptical attitude
towards applicants' stories, and address the relevant criteria to
establish (or disprove) the factual basis of such claims. This is
assured by their search for appropriate documentary evidence, by
inspecting the methods whereby such evidence is produced and assembled.

In the same way, the performance of clinical teaching depends upon
concrete displays of the efficacy of the 'investigative stance' and
procedures of the competent clinician. It is in this light therefore
that one must consider the reconstruction of the patient's case in the
course of the bedside encounter.

The practice of 'guided discovery' in students' diagnoses (as in
school science) is a version of what Bernstein has referred to as
'invisible pedagogy' (Bernstein, 1975). The distinction between
'visible' and 'invisible' pedagogies rests on the manner in which
cultural transmission and reproduction are accomplished: 'The more

implicit the manner of transmission...the more invisible the pedagogy'. Bernstein's arguments are formulated primarily in connection with varieties of preschool and infant education, but they can be extended to many other settings. One of the essential characteristics of 'invisible pedagogy', as identified by Bernstein, is that 'ideally, the teacher arranges the <u>context</u> which the child is expected to rearrange and explore'. This facet of invisible pedagogy can likewise be seen in the contrivances of bedside teaching, which also depend upon the student's 'exploration' of a largely prearranged and stage managed field of experience.

It is in the nature of invisible pedagogies that the methods of control should be 'transparent': in other words, the social mechanism of knowledge production and transmission should not themselves be made apparent and explicit. Hence the organisation and construction of legitimated knowledge pass for an organisation that is inherent in phenomena of the 'real world' under exploration and investigation. The invisible pedagogy of bedside teaching practices therefore provide a mechanism for the affirmation of the preconstituted nature of illness as an ontological entity, while the social production of disease categories remains invisible.

Hence the warrant for the clinical is constantly reaffirmed through the organised practices of bedside instruction. As Armstrong (1980) puts it:

> In the clinical years emphasis is placed on how to gain knowledge (through the process of diagnosis) as against learning particular items of knowledge. This stress on ways of creating knowledge emphasises the legitimacy of the clinical gaze and its inherent epistemology. Diagnosis is the apotheosis of such method, and whether this skill is described as 'clinical sense', 'clinical ability' or the 'art of diagnosis' the doctor is ranked according to his facility with the technique.

In thus warranting the epistemology of clinical knowledge, then, bedside instruction affirms the primacy of personal experience. It is at once the means of imparting, and the charter for, the 'clinical mentality' which Freidson (1970, p.170) captures so well:

> In having to rely so heavily upon his personal, clinical experience with concrete, individual cases...the practitioner comes essentially to rely on the authority of his own senses, independently of the general authority of tradition or science. After all, he can only act on the basis of what he himself experiences, and if his own activity seems to get results, or at least no untoward results, he is resistant to changing it on the basis of statistical or abstract considerations. He is likely to need to see or feel the case himself.

Hence the clinician becomes committed to 'his faith, his pragmatism, his subjectivism', what Freidson also calls 'a rather thoroughgoing particularism, a kind of ontological and epistemological individualism'.

This faith in the primacy of firsthand perception and personal experience leads to the clinician's certainty, in that his or her knowledge and action is unassailably warranted by this touchstone of experience. This is not to deny, of course, that medical practitioners take account of other forms and sources of information: rather, that personal knowledge is granted a special privilege. The rationale for this privilege may be conveyed by paraphrasing Foucault's comments on the 'clinical gaze' (cf. 1973, p.54): the patient's bedside has always been a place of constant, stable experience, in contrast to theories and systems, which have been in perpetual change and have masked beneath their speculation the purity of clinical evidence. The gaze thus furnishes the bedrock of certainty on which the practitioner relies.

Here, then, we see the importance of the clinic in the individual apprenticeship of the young doctor, and in the collective traditions of the medical profession. Here is reproduced its most distinctive mode of knowledge. Of course there are other contexts of medical education. I have concentrated on only one. But it is one which is of particular importance, marking as it does the medical student's first initiation into the clinical culture which lies at the heart of the profession of medicine.

9 Methodological Appendix

FINDING A WAY IN

At the outset of my research it was quite clear that it would be impractical to try to cover the entire range of the medical school; the resources and time at my disposal precluded such an approach. It was therefore necessary for me to scan the medical school in order to decide upon some point of entry into the organisation and some vantage point from which to observe the students and their training. Several possibilities presented themselves initially. The first year of the curriculum is devoted primarily to basic sciences (Chemistry, Physics and Biology) and the medical content of the syllabus appeared to be limited. The second year seemed to afford greater possibilities; in this year the more distinctively 'medical' subjects are first encountered by the students - Anatomy, Biochemistry and Physiology. This period of the curriculum did appear to offer research possibilities, and I therefore spent some time, in a very preliminary, and rather haphazard way, joining the students in Anatomy and Physiology. Of particular interest to me at this time was my access to the Anatomy dissecting rooms, where I chatted to some of the students as they worked on their cadavers. The intrinsic and personal interest of this experience was considerable. Just as the experience of the dissecting room is often taken to be a necessary baptism for the new medical student; 'it is often taken for granted that getting used to dissecting is a major problem for freshmen, the first contact with dead bodies must be a difficult, if not traumatic, experience' (Becker et al., 1961, p.102). As these authors note, it is a theme which frequently appears in fictionalised accounts of medical student life. Rosenberg (1969) described 'meeting the cadaver' as an occasion of stress among freshman medical students (see Simpson, 1972, p.66). The students I talked to in the dissecting rooms and on later occasions recounted their own misgivings and unease on first encountering their own cadaver - often with a sort of 'black humour' recounted at their own expense. There were one or two stories of students (female) being unable to go through with dissection and withdrawing from the faculty. For most of them, for most of the time, however, the experience seemed to be assimilated in a matter-of-fact manner (cf. Becker et al., 1961, p.103). Nevertheless I too took it as a personal initiation into the world of medicine. I had the half articulated notion that if the medical students had to go through the symbolic *'rite de passage'* (van Gennep, 1960) of the dissecting room, then I too should share this most salient of their experiences. Although in the event this brief period in Anatomy did not form part of the research reported here, it did on occasion stand me in good stead with the students - in establishing my *bona fides* and my credentials with them.

Despite the interest of these preliminary observations, I felt that I ought to focus my main research further on in the students' training. The students in Anatomy and Physiology were looking forward to their first contact with the work of clinical medicine, in the fourth year of the course. They saw the move from preclinical to clinical studies as a major landmark in their lives. The students' initial exposure to clinical work therefore suggested itself as a likely point for the examination of the development of students' views on the nature of medical work, and their perceptions of the various clinical specialities. My final decision, therefore, was to undertake a study of the fourth year, the first clinical year.

GETTING STARTED

Having decided that I wanted to concentrate on the first year of clinical studies, and having committed myself to the aim of doing the research by means of participant observation, I was then faced with the problem of negotiating access to the hospital wards. As it transpired, there was nothing inherently difficult in this, but it did prove a very lengthy process. My negotiations really began with the Professor of Medical Education, who was also the Executive Dean of the Medical Faculty. Had it not been for his interest and support I have no doubt that my research - at least in the form it took - would not have got off the ground. It was he who sponsored my application for permission to spend time with the students on the hospital wards. There was some problem insofar as the methodology of participant observation was rather alien to the scientific outlook of the members of the Medical School staff. Research on medical students and their education is by no means unusual, and much of the British research has been done in Edinburgh. But the research paradigms employed tend to rely heavily on the administration of attitude surveys, or personality inventories. The emphasis is very strongly on the quantitative approach to such research; my approach did not square with the normal expectations of worthwhile research, and seemed 'woolly' and 'subjective'. (Needless to say, this view is not confined to members of medical schools!)

However, in the event, a formula was found which did appear to satisfy the sensibilities of the Faculty members. The minutes of the Faculty meeting which approved my research proposal gave me permission to associate unobtrusively with groups of students, on the understanding that this would in some sense be a preliminary strategy until I formulated more detailed research proposals. In the event, once this general approval had been granted, it became apparent that such further details were not really required.

The permission granted by the Faculty also made it clear that my actual participation in medical work was dependent upon the permission of the relevant Head of Department, and of the doctors on the individual clinical units. Thus even though the initial hurdle had been cleared, I was still faced with a number of further negotiations before I could actually join the students on the wards. The Faculty of Medicine office sent out a duplicated letter from the Executive Dean, introducing me and reproducing the Faculty minute that gave me permission to go ahead.

For my first unit in medicine, I had already made contact with some of the staff members, via introductions from another member of the medical school staff. Thereafter, in order to gain access to further units I simply asked the senior consultant of each 'firm' for his permission to join his students. Although I was from time to time warned that individual consultants might prove 'difficult' and be unwilling to let me come and spend time in their wards, I was in fact refused access by only one of the consultants I approached. Since there were far more clinical units than I could cover anyway (seventeen in all), this one refusal did not in any way hamper or hold up the research as a whole.

For the most part, the chiefs of the various firms did not lay down any strong conditions on my research, and none of them subjected me to the sort of searching 'grilling' that I had rather expected. Most of them claimed that they 'vaguely remembered' the letter that had been circulated from the Faculty office. In making my requests for access I found it remarkably difficult to explain to the doctors what it was that I was planning to do on their wards. However, I found that they themselves readily translated my stumbling outline into the general formulation of 'communication' - between doctors and students, and between students and patients. I believed that this formulation of theirs adequately covered what I wanted to observe, and that in agreeing to it as a description of my research interests I was not guilty of any serious misrepresentation. This interpretation of my research project was also voiced as I did the research. For instance, during my work in medicine I noted:

> Dr McDonald then came into the teaching room. Before he began
> to teach he turned to me, and explained that the students
> would shortly be looking at case history notes, and as yet did
> not know about the normal ranges and values for haematological
> reports. He was therefore going to take a tutorial on the
> interpretation of haematology lab. reports. He went on to say
> to me that there would be 'no fancy patient-contact stuff -
> it's all meaty stuff'.

It was also a recurrent perception on the part of clinicians that I was involved in some directly evaluative exercise. It was a common reaction to take it that I was involved in action research which was directly and immediately oriented to the formulation of improved teaching practices on the clinicians' part. For example, one senior registrar in medicine confided in me that he welcomed my presence and the research I was doing. He had, he explained, been in the army and he was worried, as he felt that he could teach the assembly and maintenance of a bren gun much better than he could teach on a patient. He was worried over his own teaching, and the nature of clinical instruction in general. I tried to disabuse him of the notion that I was sufficiently expert in educational theory and methods to offer any immediate advice in this area. But other doctors would occasionally defer to me as an 'educational expert' - for instance when propounding some pet educational theory of their own to the students they would stop and seek my approval for their ideas. On such occasions I was forced to equivocate; in the context of a teaching occasion I was not able to go into any lengthy discussions of my research, its methods and its implications.

Students would likewise formulate their own interpretations of what my research might be about. The most usual solution lay in the assumption that mine was an evaluative research project. They took it that I was evaluating either clinical teaching in general, the approach of individual teachers, or both. They therefore expected me to be able to make comments on the 'efficiency' of bedside teaching as an educational method, or the nature of small-group dynamics at the bedside and in the tutorial room. Although I would try to explain that

I was not directly involved in evaluation, I was never able to convince
some of the students fully that this was the case. They tended to
assume that I was interested in their experiences on their clinical
attachments (as indeed I was) as evidence of their educational merit;
the information that students volunteered on this score served the
purpose of my developing research concerns, however, despite being based
on false premises.

However, both students and clinical staff were almost unfailingly
satisfied to leave me to my own devices - to ignore my presence when
they were busy with other things, and to talk with me when they had
time and when we had things to talk about.

DAY TO DAY NEGOTIATIONS

Although I found that it was relatively straightforward to be granted
permission to attend clinical teaching periods, this did not mean that
my day to day presence on the wards was unproblematic. Quite apart from
the senior consultants concerned, I also had to negotiate with the
various teachers who were engaged in the bedside instruction. This was
not straightforward. In the first place, I found that although chiefs
of firms would assure me that they would inform their colleagues of my
imminent arrival on their wards, this was not always done, and I would
find that after my first interview with the chief, I might go out of
his head almost immediately. Even when the doctors had been forewarned,
the news did not always filter through to all the members of the staff -
and the more junior doctors might well have been left uninformed.
Consequently, I would find that I was going in 'cold', with little or no
prior warning for the doctors concerned. Very often the arrangements
for my introduction had to be *ad hoc*, when I arrived on the wards. On
my first morning on one of my medical attachments, I noted:

> When I first went to wards___and___,I was not at all sure what
> sort of reception had been laid on for me, although I had
> already negotiated general access with the chief of the
> service. When I arrived, I found that the students were about
> to spend the first hour of the morning in individual ward work.
> As I was not entirely sure of my welcome, I stopped a passing
> doctor (whom I did not recognise) and asked him who was in
> charge of the students' work that morning. He told me to go
> and see Dr Foster, who was upstairs. I went upstairs to the
> other ward; I found the ward sister and asked for the Doctor.
> She went away, came back and asked me to wait. I had to wait
> quite some time.
>
> It appeared that Dr Foster himself was busy with his clinical
> work, and as I waited in the corridor I could see him
> bustling in and out of one of the small single rooms just
> inside the ward doors.
>
> After some ten or fifteen minutes, Dr Foster came out to
> speak to me....He seems quite affable, and told me that I
> could join the students for their ward work now if I wanted
> to. In fact I decided that it would be tactless to butt in
> in the middle of the students' history taking. (I had had
> to wait until after 10.30 to see Dr Foster.) So I hung about

in the doctors' room.

In the room I was quickly confronted with the necessity of
entering into a new introduction and negotiation. After I
had been there some minutes, one of the consultants...came
in with two housemen. Whilst I hovered in the corner, Dr
Robinson (I could read his name from his lapel badge) and
his junior staff entered into a discussion at the other
end of the room. Dr Robinson was going through a pile of
case notes and he appeared to be discussing patients with
a view to teaching on them. I could not hear all that was
being said, but I could hear Dr Robinson talking about
patients as suitable 'teaching material', and at one point
seemed to be discounting one patient for teaching purposes,
as the clinical findings were not clear enough.

When Dr Robinson had finished, he turned, looking shrewdly
in my direction and confronted me. 'Do I recognise you?'
he asked. I told him my name and indicated briefly why I
was there. I gathered from his reception of me that he
had heard of me, and he seemed quite satisfied. He seemed
at this first meeting to be a very pleasant and agreeable
doctor.

On this occasion, I was able to start 'observing' and to start my
ongoing negotiations more or less at the same time. Although I had
made detailed arrangements of when I was going to start work on the
unit with the chief, even the consultant I first met appeared to have
only the most vague impression that I was expected on the wards. I
had a similar sort of reception on my first surgical attachment. The
very first session on my first Monday morning had been taught by the
chief of the firm himself. But, as I recorded it subsequently, his
memory for my identity was remarkably short.

When the students all went off for coffee - at about 11.15,
I stayed behind, hoping to find whoever was going to teach
the next session and introduce myself to him. I therefore
hung about, and stopped the chief as he emerged from the
doctors' room. I asked if he knew who was taking the next
session, so that I could introduce myself. 'Yes', he
replied, 'Who are you?'

'Paul Atkinson'.

'Of course'. He put his arm round my shoulders and led me
into the doctors' room, where a number of the surgeons
were having their morning coffee. He introduced me very
briefly. 'This is Mr Atkinson, who is doing a survey of
surgical teaching'. Then he left me.

. . . .

I asked one of the consultants if he knew who would be
teaching the next period with the fourth year students,
and he told me that it would be Mr Jenkins. I
misinterpreted a non verbal cue from the consultant and
thought that one of the other surgeons present was the
said Mr Jenkins. Discovering my mistake (and feeling
even less at ease) I then asked if Mr Jenkins was around.

Mr Mackay said he was 'down in SCD', and that they themselves
would be going down there shortly. When he had finished his
coffee, he took me downstairs, to what turned out to be the
Surgical Consultation Department (i.e., an out patient
department). He went into one of the little consultation
rooms and brought out Mr Jenkins, whom he introduced to me,
and who readily agreed to my joining his teaching session.

It was often extremely difficult to find the doctors in order to
introduce myself to them before they came to teach the students.
Sometimes I would have short notice - or no notice at all - of who was
due to do the teaching; this was a particular problem of my first days
in a new clinical unit, when I and the students might be unsure of the
routine, and of who the various personalities involved were. When I did
find out who was due to teach, I would also find that when I tried to
contact them beforehand, they would be working at a different hospital
for the day, or were in theatre, or in clinics, or were otherwise
unobtainable. It was not unknown for me to make my first contact with a
doctor by arranging to see him between appointments in an out patient
clinic. Further, it was not always possible to predict precisely which
doctors were going to turn up to teach the students. Although some
units had a regular timetable of teaching arrangements, these
arrangements were always treated as flexible. Given the relationship
between the demands of teaching, research and patient care, the doctors
could find themselves diverted from their weekly teaching commitments
from time to time, and for alternative arrangements to be made for the
students. It could always happen that, without prior notice, the
clinique would be sent off to another specialist unit for teaching by a
doctor who was not a member of staff of the 'home' firm. In the same
way, different doctors could arrive unexpectedly in the wards to teach
the students there. For these reasons I would find myself making 'on
the spot' self introductions, and asking the doctor's permission to
stay with my group of students through his teaching period. Luckily,
despite the impromptu nature of my appearances, such hasty negotiations
were always successful, and caused no trouble with any of the clinicians
concerned. No doubt the fact that I was already clearly 'at home', and
the fact that I could always claim the authority of the chief of the
firm to vouch for my presence smoothed these potentially difficult
situations.

UNOBTRUSIVENESS AND SOCIAL RELATIONS IN THE FIELD

Although my presence on the wards had originally taken a fair amount of
negotiation, once access had been granted, I was generally taken very
much for granted by the doctors on the wards, and by the students as
they went about the hospital. I was basically left to get on with what
I wanted. Indeed, for some doctors I became so much a part of the
normal scene that they forgot who I was: I was on several occasions
taken for a student. For example:

We went to the ward, to find Dr Morrison waiting by the
entrance to the ward. He told us to hurry up, and there
was a sort of benign asperity and gruffness about his
voice. There were still some of the clinique members away
at coffee, and we stood about waiting for them. Somebody
again mentioned the graduation ceremony that had just taken

place, and the degree of BSc, Med Sci. Dr Morrison then asked
the students I was with if any of them had taken the degree.
They were mostly second year entrants and so had not done so.
Dr Morrison then turned to me and said, 'Are you a BSc Medical
Sciences?' 'No, BA Cantab', I replied. 'Oh! We should call
you Sir. What made you choose Edinburgh as your medical
school?'

I briefly reminded Dr Morrison of who I was - pointing out
that I had already been to see him to explain about my
research and to introduce myself. I told him that I had
assumed that he had recognised me again, and that I wasn't
trying to fool him in any way, or to join the group furtively.
Dr Morrison then appeared to remember who I was, and took no
further notice of me....

This interaction with Dr Morrison was not the only one in which my
presence with the students - which I thought had been registered and
taken as read by the doctor - was suddenly questioned in this way. One
such incident occurred with a physician who I had already met on more
than one occasion. He was teaching the students round the bed of a very
old lady, who was unconscious. The patient was in one of the small
single rooms which opened off the entrance to the main open ward. As
there was not a lot of room in there I tried to keep out of the way of
the students. There was in any case little to see, and there seemed no
point in my crowding in. The patient was lying on her side, with her
face turned towards the wall. At one point in the proceedings the
clinician wanted the students to get really close to the head of the bed
and observe the patient's eyes. As they all crowded into that corner, I
hung back at the foot of the bed - as I thought, being considerate.
After a moment or two the physician noticed me there, broke off what he
was saying to the students and said to me, 'You won't see very much from
down there.' Although his tone was rather sharp, I still assumed that
he realised who I was. I replied, 'Oh, it's all right, thanks, I can
see all I need to....' The doctor then made it clear that he had
misunderstood the situation, and had taken me for a student, and that my
reply sounded very inappropriate. I hastily reminded him that I was
there to observe the bedside teaching, and of who I was. 'Oh', he said,
'You're not tape recording all this, are you?' When I told him that I
was not, he seemed perfectly happy, and paid no further attention to me
throughout the rest of the teaching session.

As I have pointed out, although it was a regular part of my
negotiations for access that patients should be made aware of my
presence and the reason for my being there, such information was in fact
never vouchsafed to the patients. But from time to time I became aware
that the patients were noting my presence, and were looking at me rather
quizzically: I neither taught, nor did I ask or answer any questions.
Sometimes I did feel that I must have stuck out from the rest of the
group to some extent. However, there was only one occasion when my
presence was openly queried by a patient. It happened on a medical
unit, when my fieldwork was quite well advanced, in the third term of
the first year. I was with one of the consultants and three of the
students. The group were all seated round a patient's bed, and I sat
behind the students, towards the foot of the bed. I was visible to the
patient, but not in direct line of vision as she spoke to the rest of

the clinique. My position was, I felt, sufficiently unobtrusive, and I took some notes as the students took turns in questioning the patient. The patient herself was a middle aged woman, bright yellow with jaundice. As the students' questioning progressed, it became apparent that the woman drank heavily - and indeed that she was probably an alcoholic. Throughout the teaching session the woman's attitude towards the consultant, and to the whole exercise, was one of detached boredom - of *belle indifference*. She appeared to lack any interest in her own condition. At the same time, she did appear to feel free to pass comment on the proceedings, and to take the initiative in starting new lines of conversation (often quite alarmingly tangential to the doctor's and students' lines of inquiry). For instance,

> The patient interrupted again: 'One thing is different. I know I'm not asking the questions, but last time I had my own cutlery and crockery - which I haven't had this time - which my doctor said I should have - as it might be - what's the word?....'

Later, as the consultant and the students moved on to a discussion of possible causes and signs of obstructive jaundice, whilst they were talking amongst themselves, the patient broke in:

> 'What about the little man at the back - I can't see his face!' I shifted slightly so that she could see me a bit and gave her a little smile. Dr Maxwell and the students discussed possible clinical signs among themselves. The patient seemed quite uninterested, and was whistling quietly to herself.
>
> I took care to let her see me from time to time, making sure that I did not catch her eye too much, and so spark off new tangents in her comments.

This particular patient was rather unusual. At one point, Dr Maxwell interrupted the history taking and took the students aside to comment on how odd she was being. Her indifference and ironic detachment marked her off from the normal run of the patients I saw. When the teaching session was over, the consultant commented to me, 'She was an odd bird. She picked you up!' Of course, it is noticeable that even this patient, who asked directly who I was, hardly received a full explanation for my presence.

At times, 'unobtrusiveness' could prove rather difficult; as I have already said, at times I could be taken for a student, and 'put on the spot' by a doctor who mistook me for one. This became particularly noticeable in surgery, when I went into the theatre with the students. If we were in an open theatre, rather than behind a glass screen, we all had to put on gowns, caps and masks. With only our eyes showing it became difficult to recognise who was who - only a student's sex was apparent (and that was not always totally obvious under the voluminous theatre gowns). Under such conditions I became especially vulnerable to problems of 'mistaken identity' - I was acutely aware that I might be picked on suddenly to answer a question thrown out by the surgeon at the table. For example:

When he had removed the second part of the goitre, Mr Macdonald
said to the gallery, 'Perhaps one of you would like to go to
frozen section with it...' as he handed the bowl with it in to
the theatre porter. Mr MacDonald looked up, and suggested that
one of the two students on the end of the rows would be easiest.
Since I was sitting at the end of the row, I was one of the two.
I was by no means sure that in looking up Mr MacDonald knew who
I was, and I was very unwilling to go through any further
negotiation and explanations - either with the pathologists, or
in the presence of the theatre staff. I therefore nodded to
the other student and indicated with my head that he should be
the one to go out, whilst the group of students looked round at
each other, in some indecision. Luckily the other student went
off to take the specimen away. I am not sure whether he
recognised me either. This is obviously one of the perils of
wearing surgical masks!

WATCHING, LISTENING AND RECORDING

My periods of field observation were normally the hours of clinical work
from ten o'clock to one o'clock each day. I spent these three hours
accompanying the students on whatever activities were scheduled for
them. This allocation of time was an extremely satisfactory one from
the point of view of doing research of this sort. The morning period
was usually an active one, and required lengthy periods of concentrated
observation; the afternoon was then free to write up the notes and
observations of the mornings. This is an important consideration. The
span of memory for field observation is short and it is important that
notes should be written as soon after the event as possible - certainly
within twenty four hours (cf. Lofland, 1971). By confining the
observation to the morning's teaching I was thus able to make this
aspect of the research manageable.

In the course of the time I actually spent in the hospitals I had no
hard and fast methods of data collection. I found that my strategies
for observation and recording changed naturally as the nature of the
social scene changed. Whenever possible I attempted to make rough
notes and jottings of some sort whilst I was in the field. Such notes
were then amplified and added to later in the day when I returned to the
office. The quantity and type of on the spot recording varied across
recurrent types of situation. During 'tutorials', when one of the
doctors taught the group in a more or less formal manner, or when there
was some group discussion, and conducted in one of the teaching rooms,
then it seemed entirely natural and appropriate that I should sit among
the students with my notebook on my knee and take notes almost
continuously. At the other extreme, I clearly did not sit with my
notebook and pen whilst I was engaged in casual conversations with
students over a cup of coffee. Whereas taking notes during a University
class is a normal thing to do, taking notes during a coffee break chat
is not a normal practice. To have done so openly in the latter context
would have been to strain the day to day relationships that I had
negotiated with the students. Whilst I never pretended that everything
I saw and heard was not 'data', it would not have been feasible to make
continuous notes. As Lofland has pointed out, the practice of
participant observation must always involve a degree of 'betrayal'.

It happens that participants everywhere do and say many things
they would prefer to forget or prefer not to have known, or at
least not widely known. In the process of writing up his
notes, the observer necessarily violates these participant
preferences. (Lofland, 1971, p.108).

Such betrayal is an inescapable part of doing research of this sort,
and the collection of such 'off the cuff' remarks and observations means
that the notebook should normally remain in the pocket, to be resorted
to only afterwards.

Less clear cut was my approach to the observation and recording of
bedside teaching. On the whole I tried to position myself at the back
of the student group and make occasional jottings: main items of
information on the patients, key technical terms, and brief notes
indicating the 'shape' of the session (e.g., the sequence of topics
covered, the students who were called on to perform and so on). As I
did this over a period I discovered that a substantial amount of the
interaction could be recalled and summarised from such brief and scrappy
jottings. Schatzman and Strauss make the same point in their discussion
of field work technique:

A single word, even one merely descriptive of the dress of a
person, or a particular word uttered by someone usually is
enough to 'trip off' a string of images that afford
substantial reconstruction of the observed scene.
(Schatzman and Strauss, 1973, p.95)

During the first days of the research I found that I was producing
'filled in' field notes that were of a very general kind which described
the broad features of the action scenes I had observed. As the research
progressed, I found that I was able to observe more selectively, and
hence take more detailed notes on brief episodes of the interaction. I
was then able to spend the time in noting the direct speech on the spot,
and using the reconstruction 'after the event' to provide contexts for
these sequences of speech. On the spot note taking can never attain
the reproducibility of a tape recording of speech events, but a verbatim
account can be approximated: what is lost is usually the false starts
and hesitations that so often render totally faithful transcripts almost
unintelligible on the printed page. The field notes that I introduce
throughout the thesis, and which cite direct speech on the part of
students, doctors or patients, are taken from such notes. Where such
reconstruction of direct speech was not possible I always processed my
field notes into indirect speech, and they are reproduced in that form
in the thesis.

There is a constant problem that faces the field worker, and that is
the decision over what should be sacrificed. A complete description
would be well nigh endless, and a degree of selectivity must be
employed. To some extent during the first days in the field, one is,
willy-nilly, selective in reporting: since a great deal that happens
appears at first sight to be of little or no consequence, and its
significance is easily lost on the naive observer, then the initial
problem becomes one of finding and remembering something worth saying.
As the research progressed, I began to focus on a number of key issues,
and thus the problem of selectivity was to some extent resolved through
the development and emergence of substantive themes in the collection

and organisation of the field data.

There were some mornings when I sacrificed observation for recording. It sometimes happened that events which occurred during the first half of the morning and afterwards during the coffee break would seem 'too good to miss'. If I found that I had a great deal of action and talk that I wanted to record as quickly as possible, and in as much detail as I could, then I would sometimes stay on in the hospital canteen, and over additional cups of coffee, spend further time in writing field notes and reflecting on what had been said and done. The balance between the quantity of observation and the quality and depth of the subsequent writing is always an important and tricky element in the development of a field strategy. In the case of my own observations, I tended to proceed on the basis of a rule of thumb - and this was particularly so during the early days in the field. I would sacrifice further observation if I felt that in monitoring the morning's activities, I had made some sort of 'breakthrough'. It might be that something had happened that illuminated a series of earlier events, or which aptly illustrated some point that I was striving to understand. Such occasion thus seemed to require more immediate and detailed recording than might be the case if I postponed writing up the notes, and in the meantime confused the issue with yet more 'raw' observation. I worked on the assumption that a bird in the hand was worth two in the bush, in that one well recorded and illuminating event was worth more than two half remembered, and possibly less well reported periods of observation.

THE EXTENT OF THE OBSERVATIONS

During the first year of the research, I spent the best part of all three terms of the academic year in the field. I attended two medical units during the first term, a further two during the second term, and one more in the third term. During the second year of the research I spent the second and third terms observing surgical work. Over the spring term I attached myself to two surgical units, and in the summer term I attended an additional surgical unit.

I did not spend every available day observing in the wards: in general, I tried to spend between three and four weeks with each unit. I did attempt to put in an appearance on the wards on every day of that period, even if I was not with the students all the morning. The allocation of time was a reflection of my attempt to achieve some degree of balance between breadth and depth of coverage. As my field work got under way, it became apparent that the distinctive styles of the individual clinical units, and the contrasts between them was an emergent and dominating theme in students' discussions and their pre-occupations. I was therefore eager to sample a range of different units for myself. At the same time, it was clear that there was insufficient time to attach myself to all the available clinical firms. A period of at least a few weeks was needed to cover the activities of a firm. In some cases, there were consultants who taught only one period a week, or there were student activities that were scheduled for only one day a week. To achieve even a limited acquaintance with these aspects of the work of a clinical unit, a stay of several weeks was necessary. However, I also found that by a month of daily participation and observation, many of the features of life in the unit which had appeared distinctive were tending to become familiar, and that the freshness of my perceptions of the unit was starting to wear off. When such a sense of the familiar became apparent, I would try to move on to a new unit; by such moves I was forced to make the necessary changes in perception and understanding which threw the most routine affairs into a new relief.

By concentrating on just one year of the undergraduate medical course - a critical year, as I saw it - I was able to achieve a degree of detail and intensity of analysis that is, I believe, reflected in the resulting ethnography. Had I attempted a diachronic analysis of socialisation in the medical school, I should have had to deny myself access to the fine grain of everyday life in any of the years or locales in the medical school. Whilst larger research terms, like that of Becker and his colleagues (Becker et al. 1961), can realistically attempt more grandiose schemes of that sort, a single year's course is more suited to the one man band type of operation.

My allocation of time provided for a naturalistic sampling. My contact was mainly with the groups of students attached to the various cliniques, whose day to day experiences I was observing. Thus I was able to relate their talk (e.g., during interviews) to the social and educational context in which their experiences had been located. It was within these clinique groups that the students' consensus and disagreement over the nature of their clinical work were debated and negotiated.

ETHICS, MEDICAL AND SOCIOLOGICAL

Both the method and the subject matter of the research raised questions of ethics. My presence on the wards, insofar as I was not medically qualified or a medical student myself, was something which raised problems of professional ethics in my dealings with a number of clinicians. During the initial phases of my negotiation of access to the wards, I was informed that a few of the senior consultants had heard of my projected research and were voicing profound reservations. These were couched in terms of doubt as to whether my presence would be justified, or even permissible, in terms of the ethics of medical practice. During the preliminary negotiations with the Department of Medicine such misgivings were eventually allayed, and none of the physicians I approached withheld their general permission to join their cliniques. However, during my later negotiations with the surgeons, although general permission had been forthcoming from the Department of Clinical Surgery, one consultant, when approached, did explicitly deny me access to his wards on the basis of medical ethics. It was, he told me, contrary to his interpretation of his professional code of conduct to allow me to attend his ward rounds: he added that he found it hard to understand why the medical school should have agreed in principle to my research proposals.

More generally, the problem of medical ethics cropped up only sporadically. One consultant on a medical unit took me aside and explained to me on the first morning that I met him that he was unhappy about my presence with the students: his Hippocratic oath, he explained, permitted him to demonstrate only to those who were 'apprenticed to the art'. He added that his reservations were reinforced that morning by

virtue of the fact that he intended teaching on a female patient. On
that occasion I explained to him that I had no intention of placing him
in a difficult position and volunteered to withdraw from the morning's
teaching round. I did so with as good a grace as I could manage. It
appeared that the problem of exposing a female patient before a layman
was of more importance than the general ethical position, as I was
subsequently permitted to accompany the same consultant on teaching
rounds.

This problem of female patients provided me with some uneasiness on my
very first morning on one medical unit. When I went on to the wards
with the chief of the firm he asked me to stand some way away from the
bedside, and then drew the curtains round the patient's bed - leaving me
outside them. I could see nothing and I could hear very little of what
was going on. I was left stranded in the middle of the ward with
nothing to do but stand rather nervously by the nursing station, hoping
that nobody would come and accost me, asking what I was doing there. It
had been done without a word of explanation on the part of the physician,
and I was worried that I had not made my wishes clear to him - that he
was expecting this to be the regular pattern of my 'observations'.
After a quarter of an hour or so, the consultant and the students
emerged from behind the screens and he explained to me that they had
been examining a young woman with a difficult pregnancy. He had
therefore not wanted to embarrass her with my presence. After that
there was no question of my being excluded from his bedside teaching
sessions, or those of his colleagues on the unit. Of course, given the
nature of the work and teaching of general medicine and surgery,
gynaecological examinations were not a regular part of the bedside
instruction, and my presence was not normally a problem from this point
of view.

My relations with patients raised other questions of ethics. It was
generally part of my negotiations for access that patients should be
made aware of who I was and why I was present. This was a condition
that I agreed to, as I had no wish to engage in more covert observation
than I could avoid. However, in the event, my identity was never fully
disclosed to any of the patients whom we went to see on the wards, and I
was never explicitly introduced to them. As far as the patients were
concerned, then, I was presumably a member of the student group, or
another clinician - albeit a strangely silent one. When I joined
students for their individual work with patients, they would often
introduce me to the patient with some very vague phrase about my being
there 'to see what we're doing' - without indicating that I was not a
regular member of the hospital or medical school. Members of staff
never even volunteered such vague introductions.

To that extent, then, although I was an 'open' observer with regard to
the doctors and students, I was a 'disguised' observer with regard to
the patients. From my own point of view, this was less a deliberate
strategy, but more an exigency forced on me by the situation I was in.
There was no question that in setting up teaching situations control did
not lie with the teaching consultants, registrars or housemen. To that
extent, both the negotiation of permission to teach, and disclosure of
my identity, were the prerogative of the clinicians themselves. For me
to attempt to enter into separate negotiations, and to achieve an open
identity for myself when the clinicians remained silent, would have been
to question the position of the doctors. It could have endangered the

entire enterprise.

Just as I was a disguised observer in relation to the patients, I was in a similar position with regard to the nursing and other para-medical staff. As I mingled with the various groups of students I passed as a student myself - and I very rarely had occasion to negotiate a fresh identity with members of the nursing staff. The main occasion when I did so was on a surgical unit, when a theatre sister took an impromptu session with the students on basic surgical theatre technique (scrubbing up, putting on gloves and gowns, and so on). This fact is in itself telling. It highlights the degree of separation between the physicians and medical students on the one hand and the nursing staff on the other. There was little interaction between the two sides in the course of the clinical work that I observed in my two years in medicine and surgery. Rather, my impression was one of a relatively self contained group as clinician and students moved around the wards. It was therefore rather easy for me to pass as a taken for granted, socially 'invisible' medical student like all the others.

The problem of 'disguised' or 'secret' observation has aroused considerable controversy in the literature of participant observation (e.g., Lofland and Lejeune, 1960; Davis, 1960; Roth, 1961; Humphreys, 1970). One aspect that has been raised in this context relates to the relative power of the researcher and his 'subjects'. For instance, Davis asks himself and his colleagues:

> Is such license complete or partial? Enduring on all
> occasions, or terminal according to time, place and
> circumstances? Contingent when studying 'good' causes and
> institutions, but uninhibited when studying 'bad' ones?
> Equally applicable in whatever degree to the powerful and
> powerless alike or, as a matter of expedience, of
> differential applicability? (A colleague has ventured on
> the disquieting allegation that while sociologists are as
> a rule scrupulous in setting forth their research auspices
> and purposes when making first-hand studies of such
> powerful groups as the military, labour unions and liberal
> professions, they tend to be a good deal less conscientious
> on this score when studying such powerless groups and
> aggregates as isolated religious cults, deviants of various
> kinds and anonymous respondents at every twenty-third
> household). (Davis, 1960).

The distribution of power and authority between the various parties was in great measure a determinant of my own position in the field. But the situation was not simply a reflection of my position vis-a-vis a single aggregate of 'subjects'. Most commentators imply that in one's field work, there is a single category of persons - the 'subjects' with whom the field worker is either 'open' or 'secret'. For my part this was not the case. Not only was I concerned with staff, students and patients, but I was implicated in their power relationships. For instance, although I was 'open' with the students, once a teaching clinician had accepted me into a tutorial group, it seems extremely unlikely that the students would have presumed to question my presence. The power to grant or withhold the privilege of access to the group and its daily life was not equally shared by the students and the staff. To a considerable degree it was quite possible for the staff to 'foist' me onto their students, whilst the students had nothing like the same discretion in deciding whether I should observe their teachers. In the same way I was very largely dependent on the doctors for my identity with the patients. It was very definitely the doctors who called the tune in that situation: for me, the students and the patients. Although the others had some leeway in redefining the situation, it was the doctors who routinely defined the task and who coordinated the activities of the actors. Had I made an issue of disclosure, then it was as much my position with the doctors as that with the patients that would have been under question.

Does the fact that the patients did not know who I was mean that I arrogated to myself some privileged status as a detached and uninvolved observer, above such personal and moral questions? I do not think so. On the contrary, I believe the reverse to be true. I believe that it was rather a recognition that I was on a par with the students and the other actors, and was myself implicated in their day to day interactions. Roth (1961) has a relevant comment here:

> When we are carrying out a piece of social research involving
> the behaviour of other people, what do we tell them under
> what circumstances? Posing the question in this manner puts
> us in the same boat with physicians, social workers,
> prostitutes, policemen and others who must deal with
> information which is sometimes delicate, threatening, and
> highly confidential.

As I have tried to make clear, I was indeed 'in the same boat with physicians'. There were many occasions and many patients when the doctors did not disclose information that they had access to: in some ways, my identity was one more piece of such information. In a study which was, in part, addressed to the control and exchange of information between students, patients and doctors, what the participants did or did not do with their knowledge of my identity was itself a very revealing source of insight into dynamics of information control at the bedside.

I am not trying to moralise on this point, and on the practices of the doctors concerned. As I have shown, the creation and maintenance of a bedside interaction is not a straightforward matter. The presence of students is itself a potentially threatening one: their competence in clinical work and interactions cannot be assumed, and their participation is ambiguous, in that they are partly 'medical' people, and partly 'lay' people. The explicit addition of a totally 'lay' person could have strained the encounter to an intolerable degree for the other participants. It is part of the price that one pays for undertaking 'naturalistic' research that one's fate in the field is very largely in the hands of others. The rhetoric of 'control' is part of the language of experimental or quasi-experimental research: it is inherent in the method that the 'subjects' of experimentation, and the setting of their behaviour should be under the control of the researcher to the maximum extent. In field work, such control has to be surrendered. The 'subjects' are responsible for their own activities and for constituting the setting of the research. In my own field work I was to a great extent in the hands of the consultant doctors in matters of what I could and could not do, where I could go and so on. In this way, my relationship with the patients was almost entirely mediated by the acts of the doctors (and, occasionally, the students). My stance

of 'closed' or 'surreptitious' observation of the patient was,
therefore, not the result of my superior power (as Davis implies), but
a reflection of my inferior position. It must be borne in mind that
the status of the students was not always made clear to the patients.
Sometimes doctors would introduce them as 'a group of medical students',
sometimes as 'these young doctors'. (As I discuss below, there was some
difference in the extent to which students thought that the patients had
oriented to them as 'doctors' or 'students'). To that extent, my own
equivocal position was analogous to that of the students themselves.

Finally, it must also be added that in order to preserve the
confidentiality of my observations, and the anonymity of the staff,
students and patients concerned, all the names used in the course of the
monograph are pseudonyms. I have not attempted to disguise the identity
of all the hospitals involved - they are too well known in the context
of the Edinburgh medical school for this to be realistic. However,
there are occasions when the use of a particular hospital's name would
limit reference to a single clinical unit, and hence by implication to a
single chief of a firm. In such cases I have not referred to the
hospital by name.

Bibliography

Armstrong, D., 'Health Care and the Structure of Medical Education', in
    Noack, H. (ed), Medical Education and Primary Health Care, Croom Helm,
    London 1980.
Atkinson, P.A., 'Kind Hearts and Curettes', New Society, 27th July 1971,
    pp.178-80.
Atkinson, P.A., 'Worlds Apart: Learning Environments in Medicine and
    Surgery', British Journal of Medical Education, vol.7, 1973,pp.218-24.
Atkinson, P.A., "Centre" and "Periphery": Further Analysis of Learning
    Environments in the Edinburgh Medical School', British Journal of
    Medical Education, vol.8, 1974, pp.234-40.
Atkinson, P.A., The Clinical Experience: An Ethnography of Medical
    Education, unpublished PhD thesis, University of Edinburgh 1976.
Atkinson, P.A., 'Professional Segmentation and Students' Experience in a
    Scottish Medical School, Scottish Journal of Sociology, vol.2, 1977,
    pp.71-85.
Atkinson, P.A., 'The Reproduction of Professional Community', in
    Dingwall, R. and Lewis, P. (eds), The Sociology of the Professions:
    Lawyers, Doctors and Others, Macmillan, London, forthcoming.
Atkinson, P.A. and Delamont, S., 'Mock-Ups and Cock-Ups: The Stage-
    Management of Guided Discovery Instruction', in Woods, P. and
    Hammersley, M. (eds), School Experience, Croom Helm, London 1977.
Atkinson, P.A., Reid, M.E. and Sheldrake, P.F., 'Medical Mystique',
    Sociology of Work and Occupations, vol.4, 1977, pp.243-80.
Becker, H.S. and Geer, B., 'The Fate of Idealism in Medical School',
    American Sociological Review, vol.23, 1958, pp.50-56.
Becker, H.S. and Geer, B., 'Latent Culture: A Note on the Theory of
    Latent Social Roles', Administrative Science Quarterly, vol.5, 1960,
    pp.304-13.
Becker, H.S., Geer, B., Hughes, E.C. and Strauss, A.L., Boys in White:
    Student Culture in Medical School, University of Chicago Press,
    Chicago 1961.
Berger, P. and Luckmann, T., The Social Construction of Reality, Allen
    Lane, London 1967.
Bittner, E., 'The Concept of Organization', Social Research, vol.32,
    1965, pp.239-55.
Bucher, R. and Stelling, J.G., Becoming Professional, Sage, Beverly
    Hills 1977.
Bernstein, B., 'Class Pedagogies: Visible and Invisible', in Class,
    Codes and Control,vol.3, Routledge and Kegan Paul, London 1975.
Cartwright, A., Human Relations and Hospital Care, Routledge and Kegan
    Paul, London 1964.
Coleman, J., Katz, E. and Menzel, H., Medical Innovation: A Diffusion
    Study, Bobbs-Merrill, Indianapolis 1966.
Comrie, J.D.,History of Scottish Medicine (2 vols.) Balliere, Tindall
    and Cox, London 1932.
Crooks, J., 'Clinical Teaching in the Medical Curriculum of the
    University of Dundee', in Curriculum Changes in United Kingdom Medical
    Schools, Association for the Study of Medical Education, Dundee 1974.
Davis, F., 'Comment on "Initial Interaction of Newcomers in Alcoholics
    Anonymous"', Social Problems, vol.8, 1960, pp.364-65.

Davis, F.,'Deviance Disavowal: The Management of Strained Interaction by the Visibly Handicapped', Social Problems, vol.9, 1961, pp.120-32.

Davis, F., Passage Through Crisis, Bobbs-Merrill, Indianapolis 1963.

Davis, F., 'Professional Socialization as Subjective Experience: The Process of Doctrinal Conversion among Student Nurses', in Becker, H.S. et al. (eds), Institutions and the Person, Aldine, Chicago 1968.

Delamont, K.S., Academic Conformity Observed: Studies in the Classroom, unpublished PhD thesis, University of Edinburgh 1973.

Dingwall, R., The Social Organisation of Health Visitor Training, Croom Helm, London 1977.

Dowling, H.F. and Cotsonas, N.J., 'The Training of the Physician: Attitudes toward Patients of Full-Time and Practising Instructors as Revealed in Student Questionnaires', New England Journal of Medicine, vol.271, 1964, pp.716-18.

Eastwood, M., 'The Edinburgh of 1821', Synapse, vol.21, 1972, pp.11-14.

Ellis, J.R., 'Should the Medical Course be Shortened?' in Curriculum Changes in United Kingdom Medical Schools, Association for the Study of Medical Education, Dundee 1975.

Emerson, J.P., 'Behaviour in Private Places: Sustaining Definitions of Reality in Gynaecological Examinations', in Dreitzel, H.P. (ed), Recent Sociology, No.2: Patterns of Communicative Behaviour, Collier-Macmillan, London 1970.

Emerson, R.M. and Pollner, M., 'Policies and Practices of Psychiatric Case Selection', Sociology of Work and Occupations, vol.5, 1978, pp.75-96.

Eron, L.D., 'Effect of Medical Education on Medical Students' Attitudes', Journal of Medical Education, vol.30, 1955, pp.559-66.

Ferris, P., The Doctors, Penguin, Harmondsworth 1967.

Filmer, P., 'On Harold Garfinkel's Ethnomethodology', in Filmer, P., Phillipson, M., Silverman, D., and Walsh, D., New Directions in Sociological Theory, Collier-Macmillan, London 1972.

Flexner, A., Medical Education, A Comparative Study, Macmillan, New York 1925.

Foucault, M., The Birth of the Clinic, Tavistock, London 1973.

Fox, R., Experiment Perilous, Free Press, Glencoe 1959.

Freidson, E., Profession of Medicine, Dodd Mead, New York 1970.

Garfinkel, H., Studies in Ethnomethodology, Prentice-Hall, Englewood Cliffs 1967.

Garfinkel, H. and Sacks, H., 'On Formal Structures of Practical Actions', in McKinney, J.C. and Tiryakian, E.A. (eds), Theoretical Sociology: Perspectives and Developments, Appleton-Century-Crofts, New York 1970.

Geer, B., Haas, J., Vona, C.V., Miller, S.J., Woods, C. and Becker, H.S., 'Learning the Ropes: Situational Learning in Four Occupational Training Programs', in Deutscher, I. and Thompson, E.J. (eds), Among the People, Basic Books, New York 1968.

Glaser, B. and Strauss, A.L., 'Awareness Contexts and Social Interaction', American Sociological Review, vol.29, 1964, pp.669-79.

Glaser, B. and Strauss, A.L., Awareness of Dying, Aldine, Chicago 1965.

Goffman, E., Encounters: Two Studies in the Sociology of Interaction, Bobbs-Merrill, Indianapolis 1961.

Goffman, E., Asylums, Penguin, Harmondsworth 1968.

Goffman, E., The Presentation of Self in Everyday Life, Penguin, Harmondsworth 1971.

Goffman, E., Relations in Public, Penguin, Harmondsworth 1972.

Haas, J. and Shaffir, W., 'The Professionalization of Medical Students: Developing Competence and a Cloak of Competence', Symbolic Interaction, vol.1, 1977, pp.71-88.
Hall, O., 'The Stages of a Medical Career', American Journal of Sociology, vol.53, 1948, pp.327-36.
Hughes, E.C., Men and Their Work, Free Press, Glencoe 1958.
Humphreys, L., Tearoom Trade, Aldine, Chicago 1970.
Jamous, H. and Peloille, B., 'Professions or Self-Perpetuating System, Changes in the French University-Hospital System', in Jackson, J.A. (ed), Professions and Professionalization, Cambridge University Press, Cambridge 1970.
Kuhn, T.S., The Structure of Scientific Revolutions, University of Chicago Press, Chicago 1970.
Lofland, J., Analysing Social Settings, Wadsworth, Belmont 1971.
Lofland, J.F. and Lejeune, R.A., 'Initial Interaction of Newcomers in Alcoholics Anonymous: A Field Experiment in Class Symbols and Socialization', Social Problems, vol.8, 1960, pp.102-11.
Lief, H.I. and Fox, R.C., 'Training for "Detached Concern" in Medical Students', in Lief, H.I. et al. (eds), The Psychological Basis of Medical Practice, Harper and Row, New York 1963.
MacCannell, D., The Tourist, Macmillan, London 1977.
McHugh, P., 'The Failure of Positivism', in Douglas, J. (ed), Understanding Everyday Life, Routledge and Kegan Paul, London 1970.
Marx, K., Capital: A Critical Analysis of Capitalist Production, Foreign Languages Publishing House, Moscow 1954.
Mechanic, D., Medical Sociology, Free Press, New York 1968.
Merton, R.K., Reader, G.G. and Kendall, P.L., The Student Physician, Harvard University Press, Cambridge 1957.
Miller, S.J., Prescription for Leadership: Training for the Medical Elite, Aldine, Chicago 1970.
Newman, C., The Evolution of Medical Education in the Nineteenth Century, Oxford University Press, London 1957.
Norton, A., Drugs, Science and Society, Hodder and Stoughton, London 1969.
Olesen, V. and Whittaker, E., The Silent Dialogue: The Social Psychology of Professional Socialization, Jossey-Bass, San Francisco 1968.
Olesen, V. and Whittaker, E., 'Critical Notes on Sociological Studies of Professional Socialisation', in Jackson, J.A. (ed), Professions and Professionalisation, Cambridge University Press, Cambridge 1970.
Rees, W., 'Clinical Legal Education: An Analysis of the University of Kent Model', The Law Teacher, vol.9, 1975, pp.125-40.
Rosenberg, P., 'The Freshman Medical Student Circa 1968-69: A Dynamic Analysis', paper presented to the Eighth Annual Conference on Research in Medical Education, 1969.
Roth, J., 'Comments on "Secret Observation"', Social Problems, vol.9, pp.283-84.
Roth, J., 'Professionalism: The Sociologist's Decoy', Sociology of Work and Occupations, vol.1, 1974, pp.6-23.
Royal Commission on Medical Education, Report 1965-68, Cmnd.3569, HMSO, London 1968 (The Todd Report).
Schatzman, L. and Strauss, A.L., Field Research, Prentice-Hall, Englewood Cliffs 1973.
Shuval, J., 'From "Boy" to "Colleague": Processes of Role Transformation in Professional Socialization', Social Science and Medicine, vol.9, pp.413-20.
Silverman, D., Reading Castaneda: A Prologue to the Social Sciences, Routledge and Kegan Paul, London 1975.

Smith, D., 'The Social Construction of Documentary Reality', paper
  presented at the meeting of the Canadian Sociological and
  Anthropological Association, Queens University, Kingston, Ontario
  1973.
Stimson, G. and Webb, B., Going to See the Doctor, Routledge and Kegan
  Paul, London 1975.
Stokes, J.F., The Clinical Examination, Association for the Study of
  Medical Education, Dundee 1974.
Strauss, A.L., Schatzman, L., Ehrlich, D., Bucher, R. and Sabshin, M.,
  'The Hospital and its Negotiated Order', in Freidson, E. (ed), The
  Hospital in Modern Society, Free Press, Glencoe 1963.
Stubbs, M., 'Teaching and Talking: A Sociolinguistic Approach to
  Classroom Interaction', in Chanan, G. and Delamont, S. (eds),
  Frontiers of Classroom Research, National Foundation for Educational
  Research, Windsor 1975.
Sudnow, D., 'Normal Crimes', Social Problems, vol.12, 1965, pp.255-76.
Sudnow, D., Passing On: The Social Organization of Dying, Prentice-Hall,
  Englewood Cliffs 1967.
Templeton, B., 'Hazards of Teaching Adult Medicine at the Bedside'
  (Abstract), Journal of Medical Education, vol.42, 1967, p.278.
Turner, R., 'Some Formal Properties of Therapy Talk', in Sudnow, D.(ed),
  Studies in Social Interaction, Free Press, Glencoe 1972.
Van Gennep, A., The Rites of Passage, University of Chicago Press,
  Chicago 1960.
Wardwell, W.I., 'Limited, Marginal and Quasi-Practitioners', in Freeman,
  H.E., Levine, S. and Reeder, L.G. (eds), Handbook of Medical
  Sociology, Prentice-Hall, Englewood Cliffs 1963.
Zimmerman, D.H., Paper Work and People Work: A Study of a Public
  Assistance Agency, unpublished PhD dissertation, University of
  California, Los Angeles 1966.
Zimmerman, D.H., 'The Practicalities of Rule Use', in Douglas, J. (ed),
  Understanding Everyday Life, Routledge and Kegan Paul, London 1970.
Zimmerman, D.H., 'Fact as a Practical Accomplishment', in Turner, R.
  (ed), Ethnomethodology, Penguin, Harmondsworth 1974.